Home Care for the Client with Alzheimer's

Home Care for the Client with Alzheimer's

Jetta Lee Fuzy, RN, MS
Director of Development and Training
Health Education, Incorporated
Fort Lauderdale, Florida

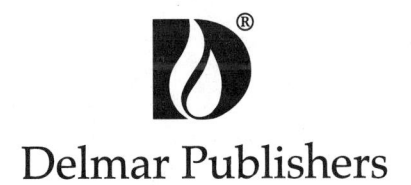

Delmar Publishers

an International Thomson Publishing company ITP

Albany • Bonn • Boston • Cincinnati • Detroit • London • Madrid
Melbourne • Mexico City • New York • Pacific Grove • Paris • San Francisco
Singapore • Tokyo • Toronto • Washington

NOTICE TO THE READER

Publisher does not warrant or guarantee any of the products described herein or perform any independent analysis in connection with any of the product information contained herein. Publisher does not assume, and expressly disclaims, any obligation to obtain and include information other than that provided to it by the manufacturer.

The reader is expressly warned to consider and adopt all safety precautions that might be indicated by the activities described herein and to avoid all potential hazards. By following the instructions contained herein, the reader willingly assumes all risks in connection with such instructions.

The publisher makes no representation or warranties of any kind, including but not limited to, the warranties of fitness for particular purpose or merchantability, nor are any such representations implied with respect to the material set forth herein, and the publisher takes no responsibility with respect to such material. The publisher shall not be liable for any special, consequential, or exemplary damages resulting, in whole or part, from the readers' use of, or reliance upon, this material.

Cover Design by Brian J. Sullivan, Essinger Design Associates

Delmar Staff
Publisher: Susan Simpfenderfer
Acquisitions Editor: Dawn Gerrain
Developmental Editor: Debra Flis
Project Editor: Elizabeth A. LaManna
Production Manager: Wendy A Troeger
Team Assistant: Sandra Bruce

Art and Design Coordinator: Vincent S. Berger
Production Coordinator: John Mickelbank
Marketing Manager: Katherine Hans
Marketing Coordinator: Glenna Stanfield
Editorial Assistant: Donna L. Leto

COPYRIGHT © 1999
By Delmar Publishers
a division of International Thomson Publishing Inc.
The ITP logo is a trademark under license.

Printed in the United States of America

For more information, contact:
Delmar Publishers
3 Columbia Circle, Box 15015
Albany, New York 12212-5015

International Thomson Publishing Europe
168–173 Berkshire House
High Holborn
London, WC1V7AA
England

Nelson ITP, Australia
102 Dodds Street
South Melbourne,
Victoria, 3205 Australia

Nelson Canada
1120 Birchmount Road
Scarborough, Ontario
M1K5G4, Canada

International Thomson Publishing France
Tour Maine-Montparnasse
33 Abenue du Maine
75755 Paris Cedex 15, France

International Thomson Editores
Seneca 53
Colonia Polanco
11560 Mexico D. F. Mexico

International Thomson Publishing GmbH
Königswinterer Strasse 418
53227 Bonn
Germany

International Thomson Publishing Asia
60 Albert Street
#15–01 Albert Complex
Singapore 189969

International Thomson Publishing—Japan
Hirakawa-cho Kyowa Building, 3F
2-2-1 Hirakawa-cho, Chiyoda-ku,
Tokyo 102, Japan

ITP Spain/Paraninfo
Calle Magallanes, 25
28015-Madric, Expana

All rights reserved. No part of this work covered by the copyright hereon my be reproduced or used in any form or by any means—graphic, electronic, or mechanical, including photocopying, recording, taping, or information storage and retrieval systems—without the written permission of the publisher.

1 2 3 4 5 6 7 8 9 10 XXX 03 02 01 00 99 98

Library of Congress Cataloging-in-Publication Data

Fuzy, Jetta Lee.
    Home care for the client with Alzheimer's / Jetta Lee Fuzy.
      p. cm.
    Includes Index.
    ISBN: 0-8273-7933-1
    1. Alzheimer's disease--Patients--Home care. 2. Home care services. 3. Home health aides. I. Title.
RC523.F89   1998
362.1'96831--dc21

98-20363
CIP

JOIN US ON THE WEB: www.DelmarAlliedHealth.com

Your Information Resource!
• What's New from Delmar • Health Science News Headlines
• Web Links to Many Related Sites
• Instructor Forum/Teaching Tips • Give Us Your Feedback
• Online Companions™
• Complete Allied Health Catalog • Software/Media Demos
• And much more!

Delmar Online To access a wide variety of Delmar products and services on the World Wide Web, point your browser to: **http://www.delmar.com/delmar.html**

A service of I(T)P®

Table of Contents

Preface vii
Introduction ix
List of Procedures xi

Chapter 1 Anatomy and Physiology of the Nervous System 1
   The Nervous System 2
   The Brain 3

Chapter 2 Memory Disorders 7
   Normal Aging 8
   Depression 9
   Delirium 10
   Senile Dementia 10

Chapter 3 Alzheimer's Disease 15
   Disease Process 16
   Three Stages of Alzheimer's Disease 18
   Caregiving Challenges 21

Chapter 4 HCA Roles and Functions 25
   Observing and Reporting 26
   Documentation 28
   HCA Care Plan 32
   HCA Visit Form 34

Chapter 5 Care of the Client with Alzheimer's Disease 39
   Communication 40
   Incontinence 44
   Sundowning 48
   Personal Hygiene 50
   Nutrition 53
   Behaviors of the Client with Alzheimer's Disease 56

Chapter 6 Procedures 59
   Skin Care 60
   Bowel and Bladder Training 64
   Catheter Care 72
   Reality Orientation 76
   Validation Therapy 78

Chapter 7 Education and Support 81
   Educating the Client with Alzheimer's Disease and the Family 82
   The Alzheimer's Association 86
   Materials for Young People 86

Chapter 8 The Caregiver 89
   Caring for the Client with Alzheimer's Disease 90
   The Caregiver 90
   Ways to Reduce Caregiver Stress 97
   Basic Techniques for Caring for the Client with AD 100
   Problem Behaviors of the Client with Alzheimer's Disease
   and Appropriate Responses 101
   Caring Techniques 105

Chapter 9 Safety and Emergencies 109
   Observing for Potential Risks 110
   Maintaining a Safe Environment in the Home 113
   Emergency Measures in Home Care 117
   Infection Control 122

Chapter 10 Abuse 129
   Six Types of Abuse 130
   Reporting Abuse 131
   Factors Contributing to Elderly Abuse 131
   Signs of Elderly Abuse 132
   Substance Abuse in the Elderly 134
   Prevention 135

Chapter 11 Psychosocial Influences 137
   The Holistic Model 138
   Family Dynamics 140
   Communication 141
   Stresses on the Elderly 142
   Confidentiality 150
   HCA Behaviors and Attitudes 153

Glossary 153

Index 159

Preface

This specialty training module is designed to train the HCA to work with clients who have Alzheimer's disease and who, for one reason or another, remain in the home. There are many aspects other than personal care involved in caring for the client with Alzheimer's disease (AD) and his or her family. When the HCA is assigned to care for the client with AD in the home, the client usually has regressed to a stage where the family can no longer assume total responsibility and the HCA's responsibility is to provide relief. It is our intention to educate the HCA with this program in order for them to understand AD, obtain increased skills in caring for this client, and acquire the self-confidence needed to provide support for both the family and the client.

With less and less medical coverage available for long-term care for cases such as AD, the need for health care workers who have additional training will increase greatly in the next decade. Some have described AD as "the disease of the century" because of the incredible emotional and physical challenge in caring for the clients. Traditionally, this illness has placed great stress on our medical system and the families involved.

Chapter 1 contains a review of the anatomy and physiology of the nervous system that focuses on the brain. Memory disorders, the signs of normal and abnormal aging, and other common disorders are covered in Chapter 2. Alzheimer's disease is discussed in Chapter 3 which focuses on its stages and characteristics.

The roles and functions of the specially trained HCA, especially observation, reporting, and recording the progression of AD in the client, is discussed in Chapter 4. Chapter 5 covers the caregiving challenges when caring for a client with AD. The procedures with which the HCA should be familiar when caring for a client with AD are discussed in Chapter 6, including skin care, bowel and bladder training, and reality and validation therapies.

Education and support for families caring for persons with AD is the focus of Chapter 7. The caregiver is very important in the management of the client with AD and Chapter 8 describes how the HCA can play a supportive role to this person, especially in times of stress. Safety and emergency situations, prevention, abuse issues, and psychosocial aspects of caring for the client with AD are the focus of the last three chapters. Key terms with which the reader should be familiar are in bold face in the margin alongside the portion of the text in which they appear.

As HCAs learn about the care of the client with AD, they in turn become the support system and care relief persons for the over-burdened families. The HCA should also become an advocate for improving the care and medical coverage of this disease in the hopes of increasing funds for research and eventually finding a cure for this serious and devastating illness.

ACKNOWLEDGMENTS

The author wishes to thank Jeleen Fuzy for her valuable input regarding both structure and content of this training manual. Without her patience and encouragement, I could not have completed this project.
The author also wishes to acknowledge the following individuals who reviewed the manuscript and provided valuable feedback.

Suellen T. Cirelli, RN, BSN
Visiting Nurse Association
Orlando, Florida

Rebecca Dierker, RN, BSN
Patient Care Services Manager
Desert Hospital Home Health
Palm Springs, California

Kathy Lalley, RN
Clinical Manager
Yakima Valley Home Health
Toppenish, Washington

Sandra O'Day, RN
Director of Clinical Services
Memorial Home Health Care
Houston, Texas

Introduction

Alzheimer's disease (pronounced alz-hi-merz) is a progressive and degenerative disease that was first medically described by Alois Alzheimer in 1907. This disease attacks the brain and causes poor thinking ability, inappropriate behavior, and a loss of memory. Alzheimer's disease (AD) at this time cannot be prevented and cannot be cured. The total cost of AD per year to our medical support systems is estimated at 90 billion dollars. The client deteriorates until eventually she or he cannot perform even the simplest of self-care activities. In the United States, approximately 40% to 70% of demenia clients older than 60 years of age live in long-term care facilities and 60% of these have AD.

AD has a gradual onset. The earliest symptom is usually confusion, which as we will discuss, may also be seen as a result of the normal aging process. AD is also characterized by symptoms of disorientation and inappropriate verbal statements. The later symptoms of AD affect both mental and physical abilities and can produce all or some of the following symptoms:

- personality changes
- behavioral changess
- poor judgment
- difficulty finding appropriate words
- difficulty finishing thoughts
- difficulty following directions
- gradual memory loss
- inability to do routine daily tasks
- impaired language skills
- loss of bodily functions

These changes occur within a different time frame for each client but the end result is always the same: clients who are unable to care for themselves and are essential helpless. AD affects four million adults in America, and is more likely to occur in the elderly. It is presently seen in an estimated 47% of those persons aged 85 or older and 18% of those between the ages of 75 and 84.

There is a serious concern when caring for client with AD because they often require twenty-four-hour attention over many years. How and where to care for Alzheimer's clients is a serious health care consideration. Caring for the client with AD is a team effort. AD care involves the family, the physician, support groups, a great deal of funding, and more recently, the home health team. Because AD affects clients from three to twenty years, it usually becomes a financial burden on the client, the family, and the insurance companies (especially Medicare and Medicaid).

There is a great deal of stress on the caregiver who lives with the client with AD because these clients require so much care and attention. Social issues arise from such stresses such as physical illnesses of the caregiver, leaving dependent clients alone in the home, and increases in adult and family abuse in these situations. Therefore, this disease is of concern to all society, not just the family caring for the client with AD.

Much attention is being given to the cost of caring for a client with AD as the United States government has a growing concern over future funding for long-term illnesses. Presently, Medicare and Medicaid do not have sufficient money to adequately care for these persons.

As the number of cases of AD continues to rise, health care givers, politicians, and the public must become more educated about this serious illness as the burden of caring for these clients rests more and more on the family caregiver and the HCA.

List of Client Care Procedures

Procedure 1	Special Skin Care and Pressure Sores
Procedure 2	Giving a Commercial Enema
Procedure 3	Training and Retraining Bowels
Procedure 4	Retraining the Bladder
Procedure 5	Caring for a Urinary Catheter
Procedure 6	Procedure for Reality Orientation

CHAPTER 1

Anatomy and Physiology of the Nervous System

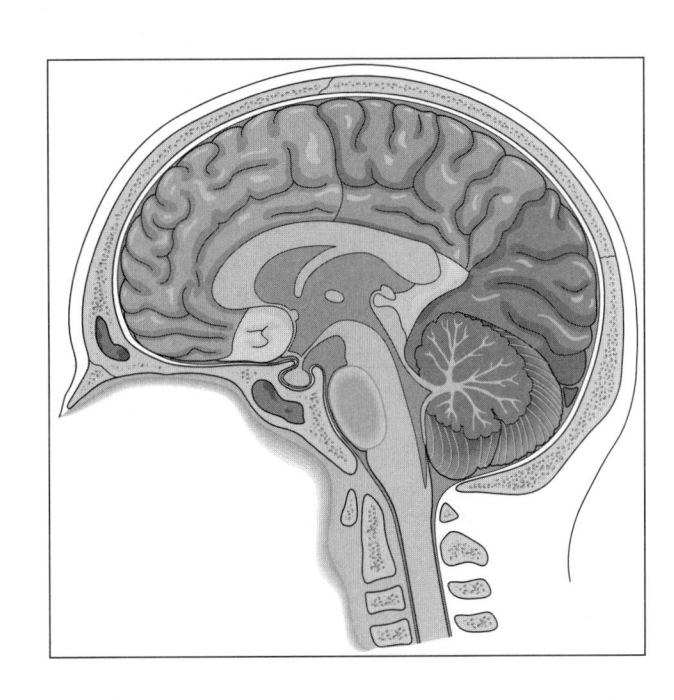

OBJECTIVES

Upon reading this chapter and completing the review questions, the home care aide should be able to:

1. Discuss the central nervous system.
2. Describe the brain and identify its five main parts.
3. List two or more physical changes in the brain tissue of Alzheimer's disease clients.

KEY TERMS

autopsy
degenerate
involuntary actions
nervous system
neurons
voluntary actions

INTRODUCTION

nervous system controls all activities of the body and has two parts, the central nervous system and the peripheral nervous system

The **nervous system** controls all the activities of the body. It has two main parts: the central nervous system (CNS), which includes the brain and the spinal cord; and the peripheral nervous system which includes the cranial and spinal nerves. The sensory organs—eyes, ears, nose, taste buds, and skin—are usually considered part of the nervous system.

neurons nerve cells which transmit nerve impulses

THE NERVOUS SYSTEM

Included in the nervous system are peripheral nerves which are found throughout the body. Figure 1–1 shows a diagram of the nervous system. Nerves are made up of cells called **neurons** which transmit nerve impulses. Nerve impulses are electrical or chemical charges transmitted through tissues, especially through nerve fibers and muscles. Figure 1–2 shows neurons transmitting messages. The impulses are sent to organs which respond or react appropriately. Neurons are protected by an insulating cover called the myelin sheath. When nerve cells are injured in the brain or spinal cord, they do not repair themselves; therefore, when there is an injury to the brain, it is necessary for another part of the brain to take over the function of the portion that has been damaged.

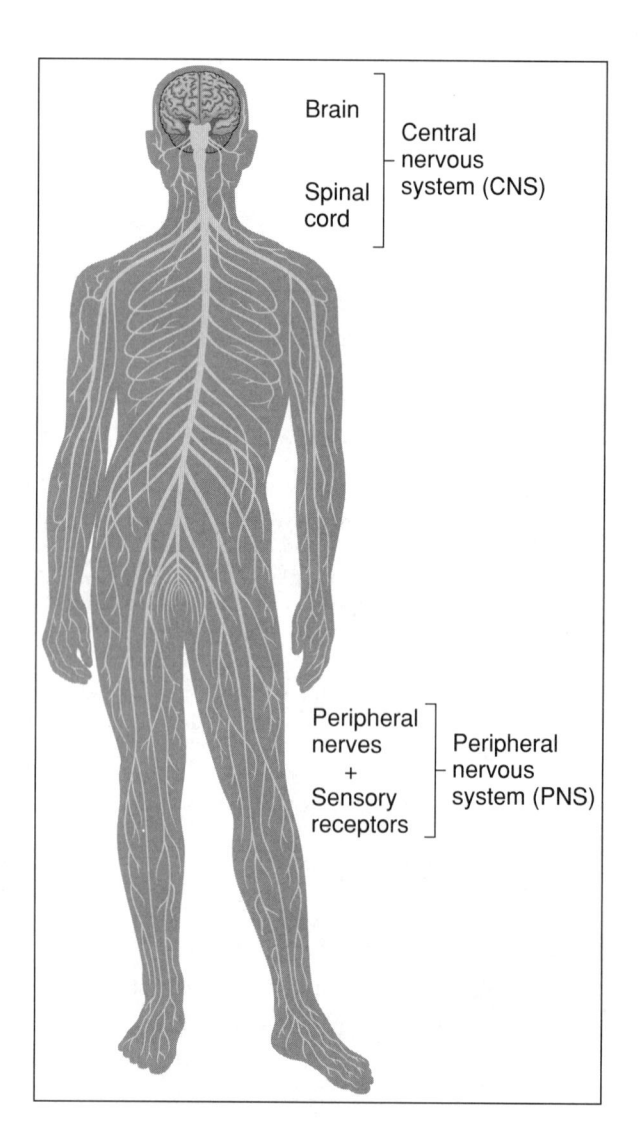

Figure 1–1 The peripheral nervous system connects the central nervous system to the various structures of the body. Messages are related from these structures back to the brain through the spinal cord.

ANATOMY AND PHYSIOLOGY OF THE NERVOUS SYSTEM   3

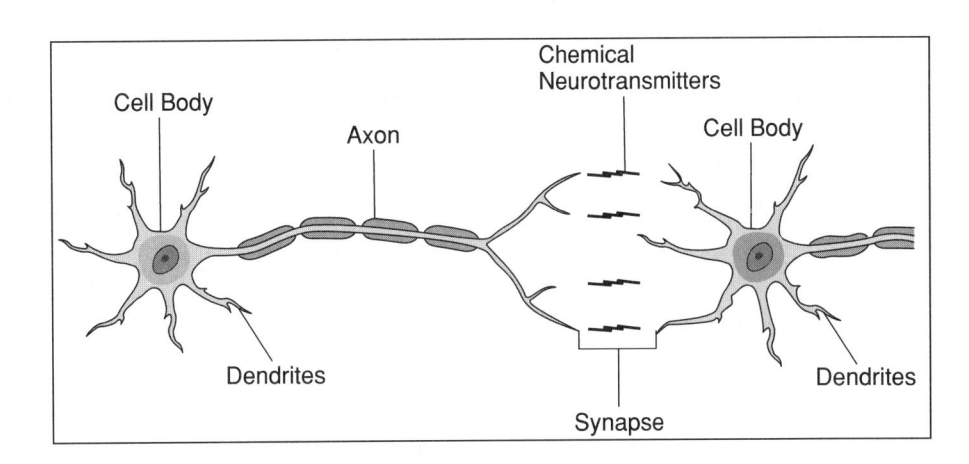

Figure 1-2 Neurons transmit messages, or nerve impulses, to other neurons.

involuntary actions breathing, heart beat and digestion all occur without a person thinking about them

voluntary actions muscular actions which are a result of a thinking process

The organs of the body usually work involuntarily. **Involuntary actions** include breathing, heartbeat, and digestion. **Voluntary actions** directed by the brain are conscious thinking processes such as walking or picking an object up off the floor.

THE BRAIN

The brain is an important and complex organ of the body. It controls every action and reaction a person experiences. Figure 1-3 shows the functions that each section of the brain controls.

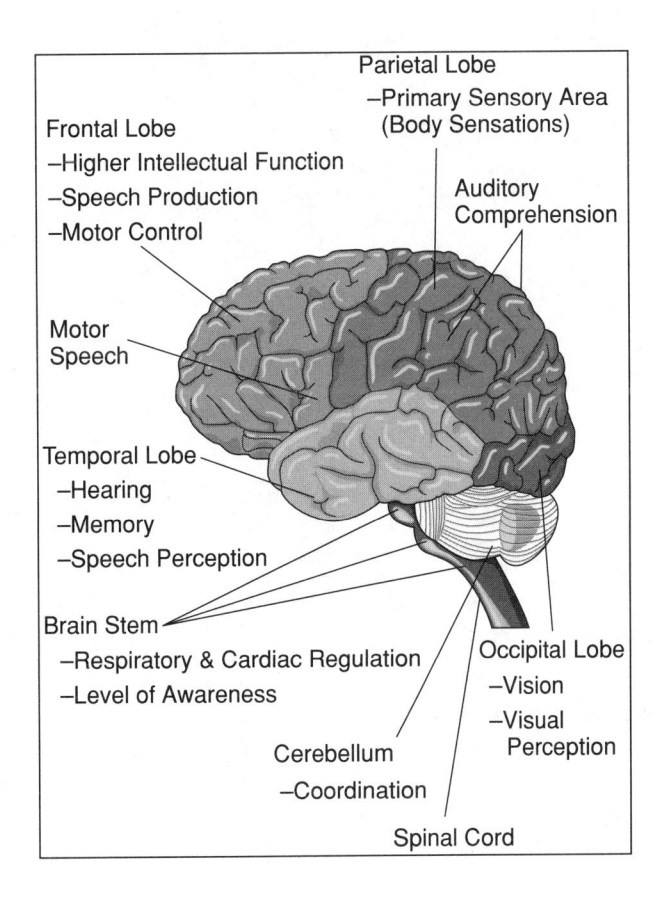

Figure 1-3 The various functions of the body controlled by specific sections of the brain.

The brain is protected by the bones of the skull and a cushion of fluid called cerebrospinal fluid. The brain has five basic parts (see Figure 1–4):

1. Cerebrum—The cerebrum is divided into a left and right hemisphere. The right hemisphere controls the activity of the left side of the body and the left hemisphere controls the activity of the right side of the body. Some of the functions located in the cerebrum are thinking, memory, emotions, and reasoning.
2. Cerebellum—The cerebellum coordinates muscular activity and balance.
3. Pons—The pons is located at the base of the brain and is considered part of the brain stem along with the medulla which controls involuntary functions such as heartbeat, breathing, and digestion.
4. Medulla—The medulla is the pathway for messages from the brain to the spinal cord. Considered part of the brain stem along with the pons, the medulla controls involuntary functions such as heartbeat, breathing, and digestion.
5. Spinal Cord—The spinal cord contains 12 pairs of cranial nerves and 32 pairs of spinal nerves whose branches go to all

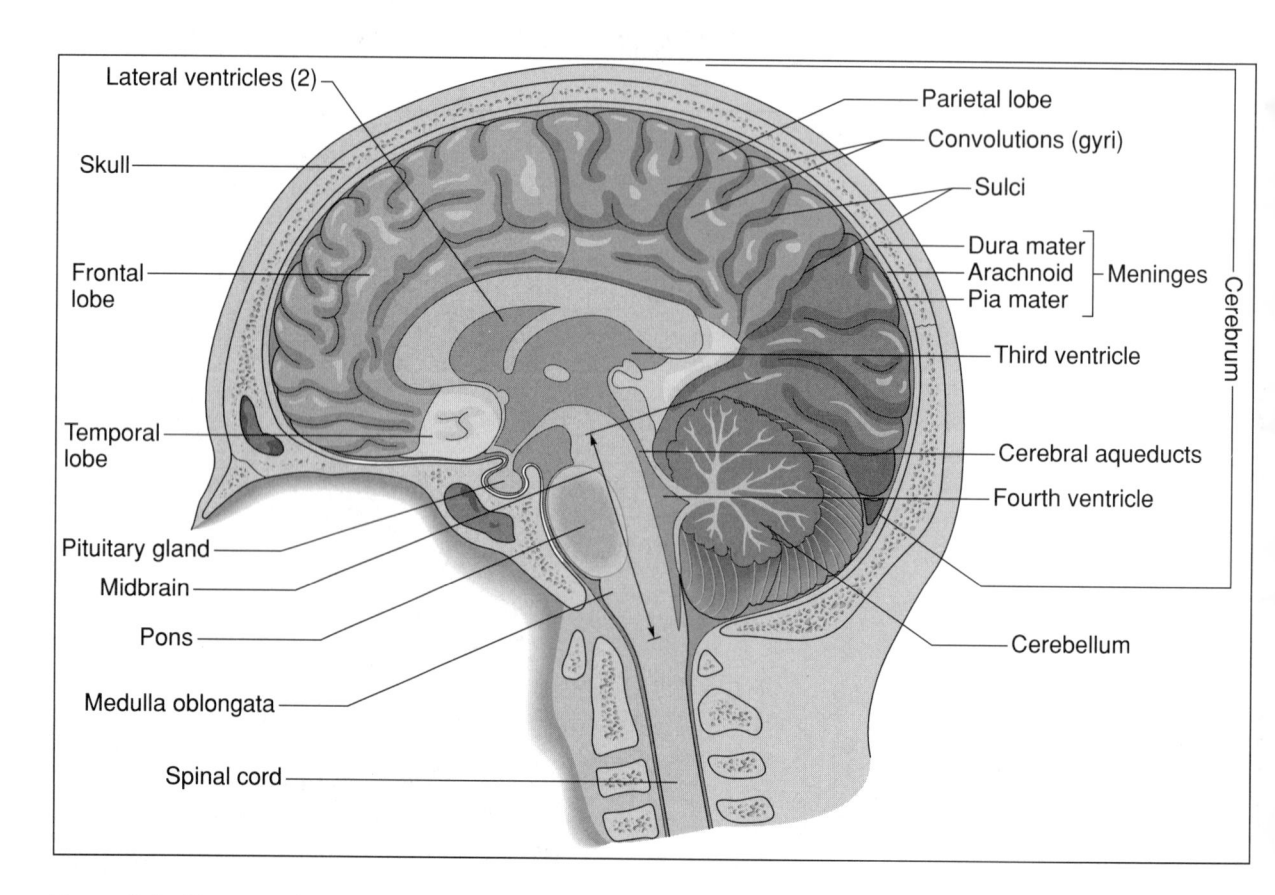

Figure 1-4 The central nervous system—brain and spinal cord.

ANATOMY AND PHYSIOLOGY OF THE NERVOUS SYSTEM   5

parts of the body. The nerves act as the highways through which the messages from the brain travel to the various parts of the body. The spinal cord is protected by spinal vertebrae and cerebrospinal fluid.

Because Alzheimer's disease (AD) affects the brain and not the spinal cord, changes only occur in nerve cells in the outer layer of the brain. A definitive diagnosis of AD can only be made upon examination of brain tissue at the time of **autopsy**. In living patients, however, the diagnostic process includes a complete physical, a neurological workup, a psychiatric assessment, and laboratory tests including a brain scan. A probable diagnosis of AD is accurate in 80% to 90% of cases. Physicians are careful not to diagnose AD in a person unless they are fairly certain of the presence of the disease because of the family's natural concern about the future of their loved one.

Microscopic examinations of the brain tissue of the client with AD shows myelin plaques and neurofibrillary tangles, especially in areas of the brain responsible for memory and intellectual function. The person with AD has brain tissue which lacks the chemical acetylcholine, necessary for the brain to process memory. The neurotransmitters, the brain's relay stations that transmit impulses from one cell to another, **degenerate** with AD. At the present time, research has not demonstrated how or why this degenerative process occurs.

autopsy   tissue examination after death

Helpful Hints: The HCA should never label a client as having Alzheimer's disease until the physician does so first.

degenerate   deteriorate or ruin permanently

REVIEW QUESTIONS

1. The two main parts of the central nervous system are the _____ and the _____ _____.
2. _____ transmit nerve impulses.
3. The five main parts of the brain are:
    a.
    b.
    c
    d.
    e.
4. The cerebrum controls:
    a. thinking
    b. emotions
    c. reasoning
    d. all of the above

5. The medulla controls:
    a. heartbeat and breathing
    b. heartbeat and walking
    c. breathing and lifting
    d. all muscle activity
6. True or False? Diagnosis of AD can only be made upon examination of the brain tissue at autopsy.
7. True or False? Microscopic examinations of the brain tissue of the client with AD shows senile plaques and neurofibrillary tangles, especially in the areas of the brain responsible for memory and intellectual function.

Match the function in the left column to the brain part in the right column.

8. _____ Cerebrum   a. memory
9. _____ Cerebellum   b. heartbeat
10. _____ Medulla   c. balance
11. _____ Pons   d. allows message to travel to organ
12. _____ Spinal Cord   e. digestion
13. Unscramble the following key term from the chapter: yatvuoilrnn snicacto _____ _____

CHAPTER 2

Memory Disorders

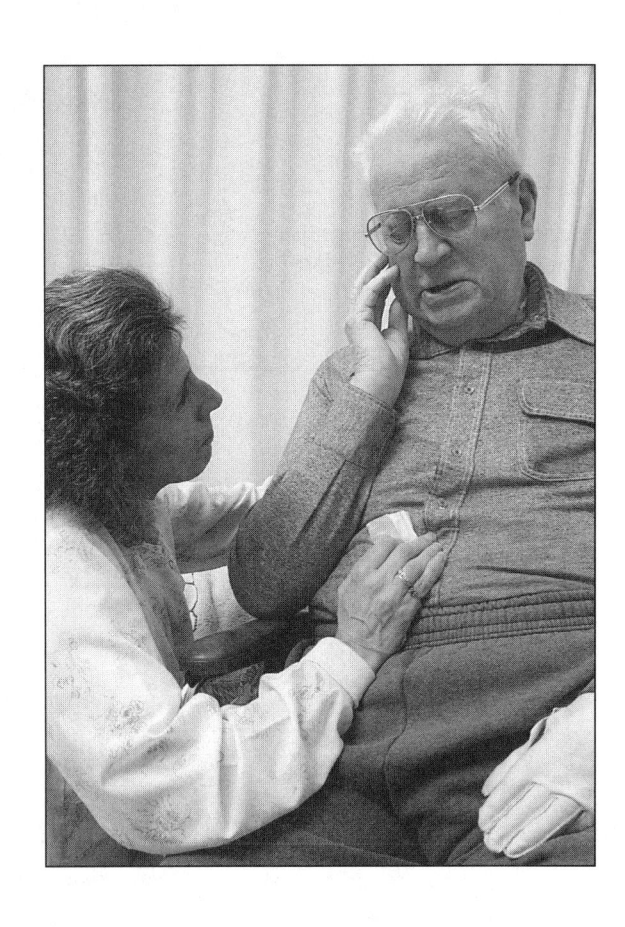

OBJECTIVES

Upon reading this chapter and completing the review questions, the home care aide should be able to:
1. Recognize the physical, emotional, and psychological signs of normal aging.
2. Define the memory disorders of depression, delirium, and senile dementia.
3. Describe Alzheimer's disease in relation to memory disorders.

KEY TERMS

Alzheimer's disease
delirium
dementia
depression

geriatric
irreversible
senility

INTRODUCTION

Alzheimer's disease the main form of senile dementia

Recognizing **Alzheimer's disease** in its early stages is difficult because the early symptoms associated with the disease are similar to characteristics of the normal aging process and of other disorders. It is important for the HCA to understand normal aging and memory disorders such as depression, delirium, and senile dementia which includes Alzheimer's disease.

NORMAL AGING VERSUS ABNORMAL AGING

senility older term for forgetfulness

dementia newer term for group of symptoms referring to a gradual decrease in mental powers and intellectual functions

Senility is an outdated, inaccurate term that was used to refer to an older person who became forgetful and who was not able to care for himself or herself. The term **dementia** refers to a gradual decrease in a person's mental powers and intellectual function and is not a normal part of the aging process. Dementia is not a disease but is a group of symptoms with various causes.

The physical signs of normal aging include the following:
- slower reflexes
- less efficient circulation
- gray or white hair
- slower bodily functions
- loss of skin elasticity
- diminished eyesight
- diminished hearing
- stooped posture
- lessened muscle strength
- lessened sensation to heat and cold
- poor healing powers
- clouding of the lenses of the eyes (cataracts)
- decreased immune functions

Figure 2-1 shows the physical signs of aging.

Mental changes in the normal aging process include the following:
- slowed reaction time
- slightly slower memory input

geriatrics the branch of medicine that treats all problems and conditions pertaining to old age

There are many emotional and psychological factors in a person over sixty-five that impact the **geriatric's** mental process. These might include:
- a change in living style
- a change in financial status
- the death of a spouse (loneliness)
- a feeling of uselessness
- a fear of dependency

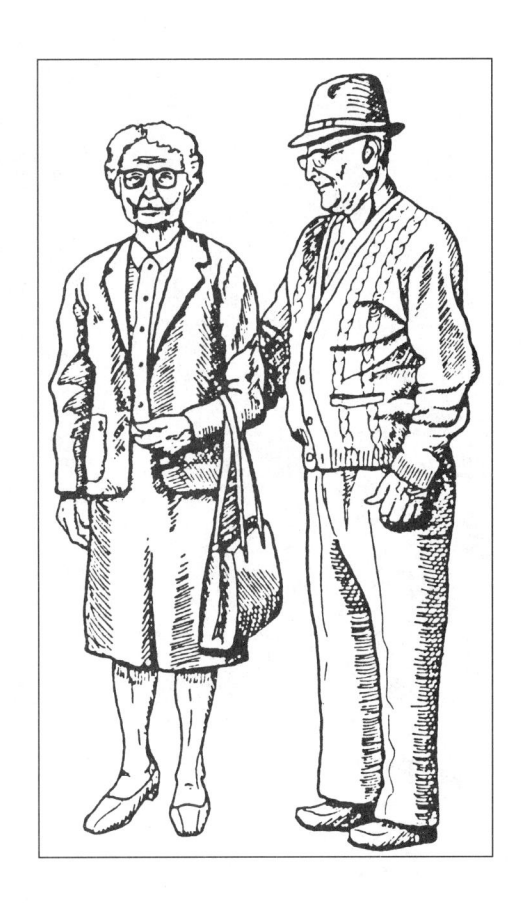

Figure 2–1 Changes in the body over time (Reprinted by permission of *Aging in America* by Sandra Zims, copyright 1987 by Delmar Publishers, Inc.)

Helpful Hints: Older clients need to be constantly assured that they are not a burden and that the HCA wants to care for them.

depression psychiatric disorder of sadness and hopelessness

Helpful Hints: Any sign of depression in the client should be reported to the supervisor so that the physician can be kept informed and a medical social worker be assigned to the case.

- alcohol and substance abuse
- depression related to multiple life changes
- poor nutrition
- illness, especially if chronic and debilitating

DEPRESSION

Depression is a psychiatric disorder characterized by sadness, inactivity, hopelessness, poor concentration and poor attention. Both dementia and depression are diagnosed in an elderly client and it is often difficult to tell the difference. Often, depression is treated with anti-depressant drugs and when symptoms are relieved, it is easily differentiated from senile dementia. Stress in the elderly, brought on by aging and changes in lifestyle, are underlying factors in depression. Treatment for elderly persons with depression includes stress management therapy. The onset of clinical depression involves insomnia, panic attacks, and phobias. Depression can also be linked to an event, such as the loss of a job, loss of a loved one, retirement, change in residence, or financial loss. Figure 2–2 shows an elderly person who is depressed.

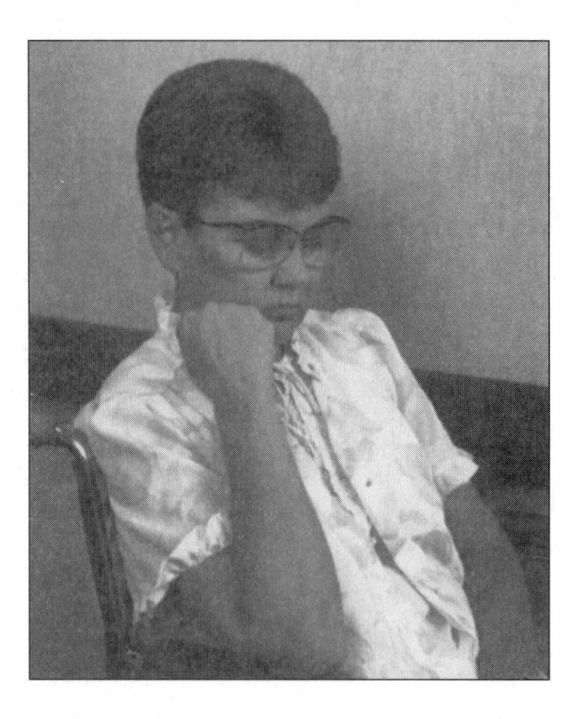

Figure 2–2 The elderly sometimes suffer from depression.

delirium physical condition of short duration with symptoms similar to dementia and/or depression

DELIRIUM

Delirium is caused by a physical problem and has symptoms similar to those of depression and dementia. Delirium, however, has a physiologic cause such as hyperglycemia, electrolyte imbalance, an embolism, head trauma, a systemic infection, or drug toxicity. Delirium has a rapid onset, and when treated, has a short duration, usually lasting no more than a few days or a few hours. Alleviate the cause and the symptoms of delirium are relieved.

The symptoms of delirium include:

- poor thought processes
- inappropriate behavior
- memory loss
- abrupt personality changes
- loss of appetite
- sleep disturbance
- speech problems
- occasional hearing and vision loss

SENILE DEMENTIA

Senile dementia is a group of symptoms characterized by a loss of a previous level of intellectual function that interferes with activities of daily functioning. Table 2–1 shows the different types of dementia. Current research shows that the cause of over half of all senile dementia is Alzheimer's disease. It is important, once the symptoms of senile dementia occur, that the cause be determined so that are treatable conditions are addressed.

Table 2–1	Descriptions of the Major Forms of Dementia	
Disease	Features	Course
Alzheimer's	Lack of chemical in brain causing neurofibrillary tangles, neuritic plaques	Onset age: 60–80 Slowly progressive
Multi-infarct dementia	Interference with blood circulation in brain cells due to arteriosclerosis and/or Atherosclerosis	Onset age: 55–70 Outcome depends on rate of damage to brain cells
Huntington's	Inherited from either parent who has gene for the disease	Onset age: 25–45 Average duration is 15 years
Parkinson's	Deficiency of chemical in brain (dopamine)	Onset age: 55–60 Several years duration
Creutzfeldt-Jacob	Nonimflammatory virus, changes in brain	Onset age: 50–60 Rapidly progressive
Syphilis	Spirochete (bacteria) causes brain damage	Occurs 15–20 years after primary infection
AIDS dementia	HIV-1 infection	Symptoms sometimes precede diagnosis of AIDS

Dementia is generally diagnosed when there is a significant deterioration in three of the following eight areas:

1. cognitive thinking
2. memory
3. language usage
4. recognition
5. reasoning
6. visual loss
7. behavioral changes
8. personality changes

Figure 2–3 shows a client with dementia.

There are four common causes of dementia in the elderly that often can be treated and successfully reversed. These are:

1. Medication problems
2. Thyroid conditions
3. Tumors in the central nervous system
4. Depression

Helpful Hints: The HCA should report to the supervisor if he or she suspects that the client is taking a new medication that is causing changes in his or her behavior.

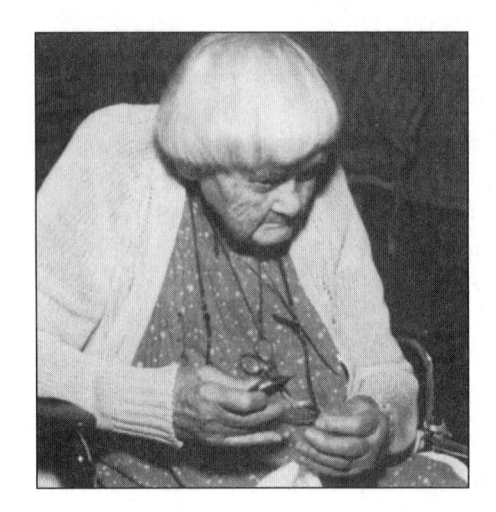

Figure 2–3 The person with dementia is cognitively impaired.

irreversible

The most common **irreversible** type of dementia is Alzheimer's disease which is present in as many as 65% to 75% of all dementia clients. Figure 2–4 shows the percentage breakdown for common causes of senile dementia.

Symptoms of senile dementia can be affected by alcoholism, heart disease, psychiatric disorders, impaired kidney function, neurological disorders, brain disorders (tumors, for example) head injuries, nutritional deficiencies, AIDS, infections such as meningitis, and Parkinson's disease. Figure 2–5 shows two HCAs helping a dementia client with exercise.

Alzhiemer's disease is the most common form of nontreatable and irreversible dementia. All persons with symptoms of dementia should be considered possible clients with Alzheimer's disease.

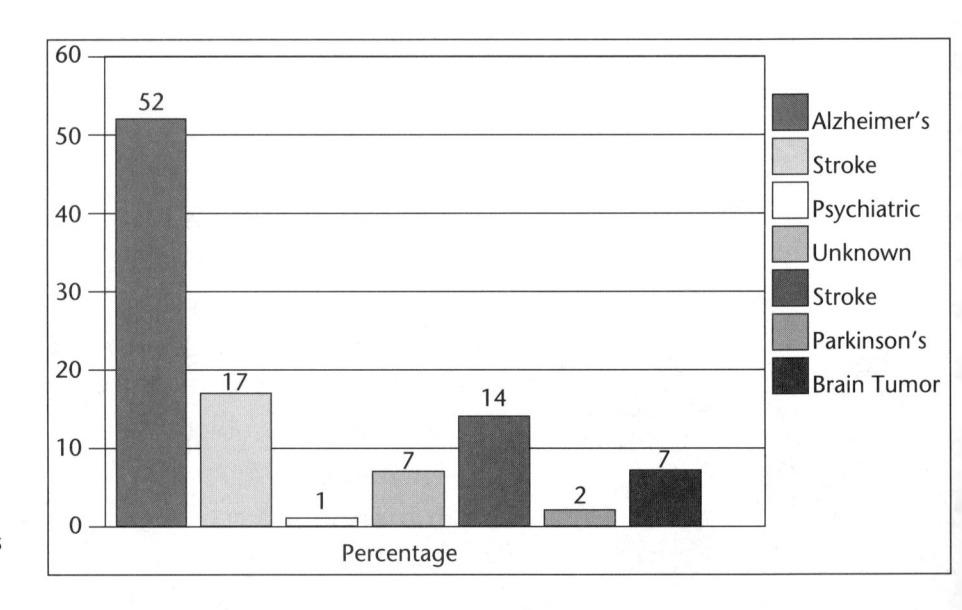

Figure 2–4 The graph shows causes by percentage of senile dementia.

Cause	Percentage
Alzheimer's	52
Stroke	17
Psychiatric	1
Unknown	7
Stroke	14
Parkinson's	2
Brain Tumor	7

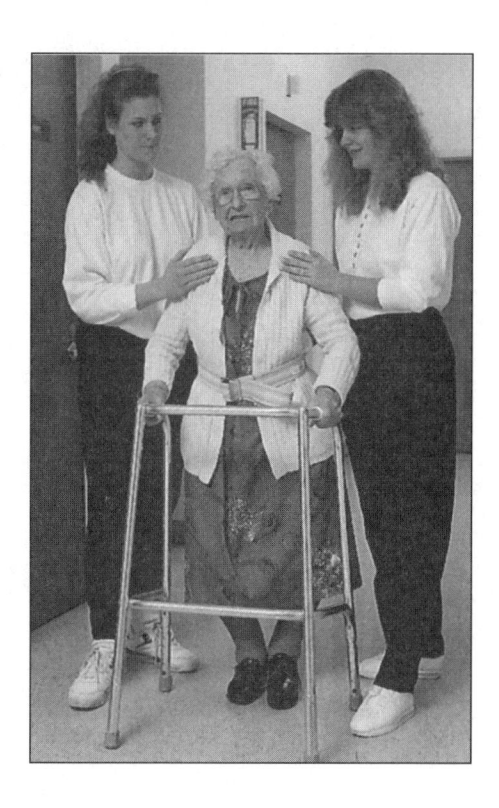

Figure 2–5 Clients with dementia need daily exercise.

REVIEW QUESTIONS

1. The term _____ means an older person who becomes forgetful.
2. _____ is a gradual decrease in a person's mental powers and intellectual function.
3. _____ _____ is the main form of the above.
4. Which of the following is a process of normal aging:
   a. slower reflexes
   b. slower body functions
   c. poor healing powers
   d. all of the above
5. Which of the following does not usually impact a normal aging process?
   a. change in finances
   b. nutrition
   c. alcohol
   d. loss of hair
6. True or False? Depression can easily be diagnosed as dementia in the elderly.
7. True or False? Delirium is common in the elderly and is often a long-term condition.

14 CHAPTER 2

8. True or False? Symptoms of a stroke may imitate senile dementia symptoms or visa versa.
9. True or False? All persons with symptoms of dementia should be considered possible candidates for Alzheimer's Disease.
10. List four causes of dementia that can often be treated and reversed:
    a.
    b.
    c.
    d
11. Unscramble the following key term from the chapter: tacregiir _____

CHAPTER 3

Alzheimer's Disease

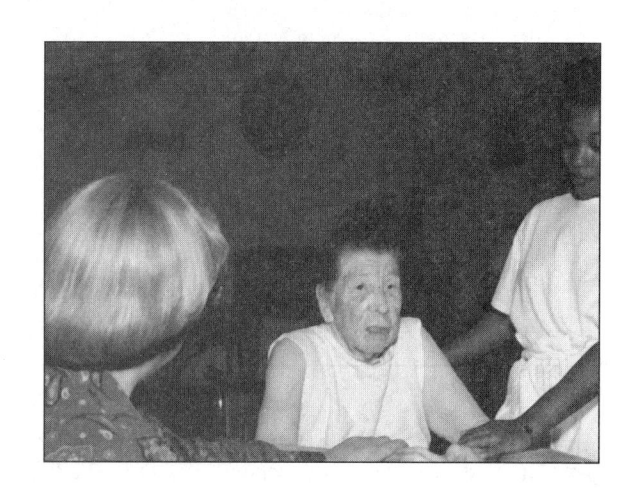

OBJECTIVES

Upon reading this chapter and completing the review questions, the home care aide should be able to:
1. Describe the disease process of Alzheimer's disease.
2. Define the two forms of Alzheimer's disease.
3. Describe the three stages of Alzheimer's disease and their characteristics.

KEY TERMS

emaciation
genetics
incontinence
muteness
paranoia
sundowning

INTRODUCTION

One out of every three Americans will be affected by Alzheimer's disease. Either a family member will develop the disease or they will develop AD themselves. It is important that research be continued so that we can learn as much as possible about this disease. This chapter discusses AD and its effects on the client and his or her family.

DISEASE PROCESS

Alzheimer's disease affects all sexes, races, and socioeconomic groups. It does not discriminate. In the past decade, increased public awareness and education has resulted in better funding and research into AD and Alzheimer's Disease Related Disorders (ADRD). ADRD is a broad term that includes disorders and symptoms associated with AD that can be treated and managed. These include:

- dementia symptoms
- all physical deteriorations
- problem behaviors
- psychological or psychiatric disorders
- functional decline
- safety concerns
- nutritional disorders

genetics study of diseases in terms of being inherited or passed from one generation to another

The cause of AD is unknown. However, recent research has pointed to the possibility of two types of AD: **genetic** and nongenetic. At this time, science has not identified the risk factors or indicators for inheriting AD and there is no evidence to prove that one person is more likely to develop the disease than another, even in families of AD clients. One type of AD, however, appears to be familial.

Because AD is incurable and is irreversible, the focus today is on the ADRDs and the management of the disease. This includes care at home or in facilities, and above all else, helping the person or persons caring for these clients.

In addition to genetic and nongenetic types, there are two other forms of AD termed benign and malignant. Benign AD is the most common form and is characterized by symptoms similar to senility such as a slow, gradual loss of memory, late-stage motor function loss, and deterioration of the frontal lobe of the brain. Malignant AD is less common and is characterized by loss of motor function early in the disease, severe weight loss, and rapid deterioration of the client. Malignant AD also shows widespread degeneration of brain tissue.

The diagnosis of AD can be confirmed only when a brain tissue biopsy is done during an autopsy. Tentative diagnosing, however, is done by interviewing and assessing the client with psychological testing, computed tomography (CT) scans, electroencephalograms (EEGs), and complete physical, neurological, and psychiatric workups. Usually, the physician rules out other causes of dementia with a complete neurological and psychiatric evaluation. Early diagnosis is important so that the client and family can be educated to prepare for the problems that arise in the later stages of AD. Figure 3–1 shows the warning signs of a person who might have AD.

Ten Warning Signs of Alzheimer's Disease

To help you know what warning signs to look for, the Alzheimer's Association has developed a checklist of common symptoms (some of them also may apply to other dementing illnesses). Review the list and check the symptoms that concern you. If you notice several symptoms, the individual with the symptoms should see a physician for a complete examination.

1. **Memory Loss That Affects Job Skills**

   It's normal to occasionally forget assignments, colleagues' names, or a business associate's telephone number and remember them later. Those with a dementia, such as Alzheimer's disease, may forget things more often, and not remember them later.

2. **Difficulty Performing Familiar Tasks**

   Busy people can be so distracted from time to time that they may leave the carrots on the stove and only remember to serve them at the end of the meal. People with Alzheimer's disease could prepare a meal and not only forget to serve it, but also forget they made it.

3. **Problems with Language**

   Everyone has trouble finding the right word sometimes, but a person with Alzheimer's disease may forget simple words or substitute inappropriate words, making his or her sentence incomprehensible.

4. **Disorientation of Time and Place**

   It's normal to forget the day of the week or your destination for a moment. But people with Alzheimer's disease can become lost on their own street, not knowing where they are, how they got there or how to get back home.

5. **Poor or Decreased Judgment**

   People can become so immersed in an activity that they temporarily forget the child they're watching. People with Alzheimer's disease could forget entirely the child under their care. They may also dress inappropriately, wearing several shirts or blouses.

6. **Problems with Abstract Thinking**

   Balancing a checkbook may be disconcerting when the task is more complicated than usual. Someone with Alzheimer's disease could forget completely what the numbers are and what needs to be done with them.

7. **Misplacing Things**

   Anyone can temporarily misplace a wallet or keys. A person with Alzheimer's disease may put things in inappropriate places: an iron in the freezer, or a wristwatch in the sugar bowl.

8. **Changes in Mood or Behavior**

   Everyone becomes sad or moody from time to time. Someone with Alzheimer's disease can exhibit rapid mood swings—from calm to tears to anger—for no apparent reason.

9. **Changes in Personality**

   People's personalities ordinarily change somewhat with age. But a person with Alzheimer's disease can change drastically, becoming extremely confused, suspicious, or fearful.

10. **Loss of Initiative**

    It's normal to tire of housework, business activities, or social obligations, but most people regain their initiative. The person with Alzheimer's disease may become very passive and require cues and prompting to become involved.

(Courtesy of The Alzheimer's Association)

Figure 3–1 Ten warning signs of Alzheimer's disease. (Reprinted with permission from Alzheimer's Association, Inc., © 1995, 1996.)

THREE STAGES OF AD

There are three stages of AD which the client goes through. HCAs should be familiar with the level their clients are in so that the care plan and activities of daily living (ADL) can be altered to the appropriate stage. The three stages of AD are discussed below.

Stage I

Stage I is moderate and characterized by forgetfulness, impairment in judgment, an increasing inability to handle routine tasks, and an increase in disorientation as to time and place. This stage includes depression, fear, and an increased anxiety level. The HCA can expect the Alzheimer's client in this stage to have the following problems:

- difficulty in selecting clothing (the client will wear the same thing every day)
- problems in driving
- weight loss of ten pounds or more
- wandering from the home and forgetting how to get back (**sundowning**)
- severe memory lapses relating to telephone numbers, addresses, dates, or the year (memory lapses change by the hour).
- withdrawn, angry, suspicious, and tearful.

Stage II

Stage II is moderately severe and characterized by the client's forgetting the activities of daily living such as bathing, toileting, and dressing, inability to understand the world around them, and the client becoming agitated, hostile, and even violent. These clients have the following problems:

Helpful Hints: The HCA should explain the three stages of AD to the client's family so they will be able to anticipate changes in his or her behavior. Figure 3–2 shows a client with stage I AD.

sundowning symptom of AD in which clients tend to wander at dark

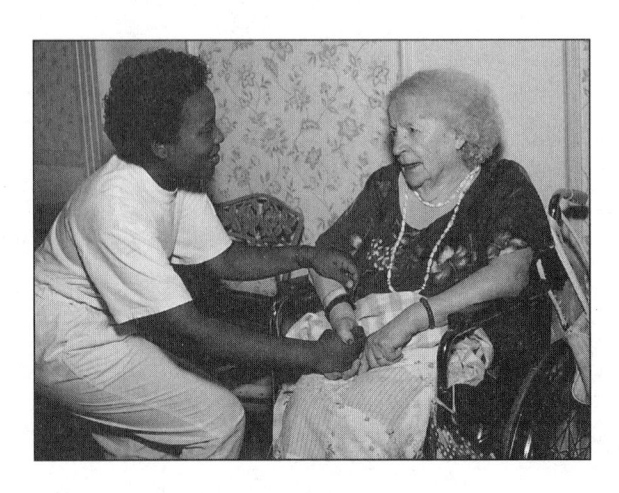

Figure 3–2 In stage I of Alzheimer's disease, the client will show some memory lapse and anger.

ALZHEIMER'S DISEASE 19

- increased memory loss (can no longer remember the family members or the HCA from hour to hour)
- inability to speak in sentences and verbalize their needs
- slow walk or movement
- fear of bathing or showering
- **paranoia** or delusions such as talking to imaginary people; extreme hostility
- **incontinence** once or twice a week
- wander and generally restless, especially at night
- muscle twitching and convulsions
- progressive disorientation

Figure 3–3 shows a client with stage II AD.

Stage III

Stage III is severe and characterized by a client completely dependent on another person for care. These client's cannot walk or perform any activity on their own. Severe AD is characterized by complete disorientation, **emaciation** (severe weight loss), and complete loss of control of all bodily functions.

The problems associated with severe AD include:

- speech impairments or complete **muteness**
- inability to speak more than one or two words, grunting, or screaming
- less agitation but less awareness of surroundings
- loss of the ability to chew; infantile in behavior and ability
- bedridden clients in need of twenty-four hour care for the rest of their lives

Figure 3–4 shows a client with stage III AD.

paranoia unreal feelings that others are "against" you or will harm you

incontinence lack of control of bladder or bowels

emaciation extreme thinness

muteness inability to speak

Helpful Hints: When the client is in Stage III of AD, the family will no longer be able to care for the client without outside help. Home health care will be needed.

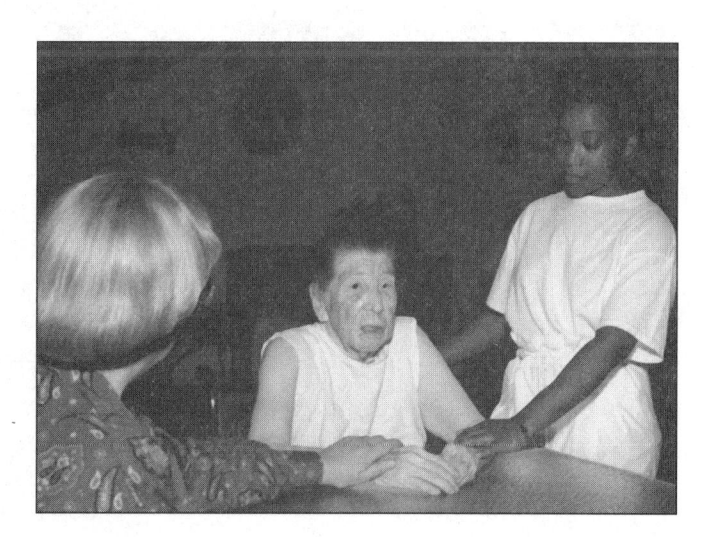

Figure 3–3 In stage II of Alzheimer's disease, the client will show an inability to understand the world around them.

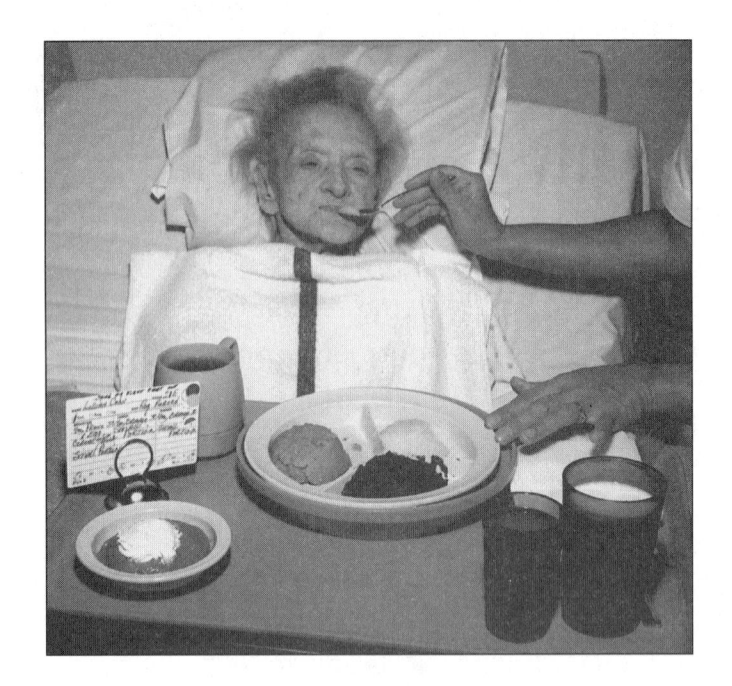

Figure 3–4 In stage III of Alzheimer's disease, the client cannot perform any function and is bedridden.

Helpful Hints: Clients in Stage III AD might have to be placed in facilities such as nursing homes to receive the care they need. Figure 3–5 shows an Alzheimer's Unit in a nursing home.

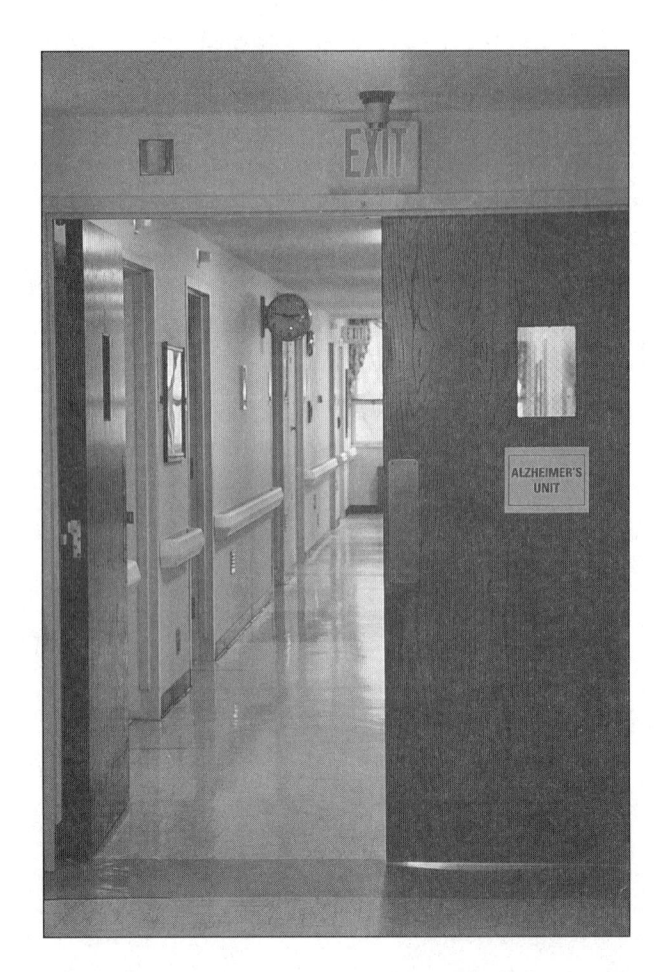

Figure 3–5 The Alzheimer's unit at a nursing home may be where many clients who are in Stage III reside.

The stages of AD overlap as the disease progresses and most clients with AD die of pneumonia, stroke, or acute functional decline.

CAREGIVING CHALLENGES

Care of the client with AD at any stage of the illness is a great challenge. The HCA who chooses to care for these clients in the home should keep two goals in mind:

1. Understand the client and his/her condition so that appropriate care is given.
2. Observe the home situation, especially in terms of the primary caregiver, if that person is other than the HCA.

Four objectives for HCAs working with clients with AD and their families include the following:

1. To provide personal care and home maintenance for the client who is living independently whether at home or in a facility.
2. To promote as much self-care, dignity, safety, and independence as possible and to consider each client as an individual case.
3. To provide relief to family members by caring for the client with an understanding of the great responsibility of the caregivers.
4. To encourage the family members and caregivers to care for themselves by knowing they must conserve their energy and manage their stress.

Table 3–1 shows problem behaviors of the client with AD and possible solutions.

Table 3-1 Problem Behaviors and Possible Solutions

Problem Behaviors	Possible Solutions
1. Unable to recognize own face or a family member's face	Use memory crutches such as pictures for self-identification and recognition of others Repeat the family member's name frequently
2. Touching and examining objects with the mouth	Make the environment safe Keep dangerous objects away from the patient Distract the patient Do not accept the behavior
3. Touching everything	Make the environment safe If possible, let them touch items which are easily rearranged Distract the patient
4. Dependent behavior when it is exemplified by insecurity and loss of control	A consistent caregiver who is warm and compassionate
5. Increased libido	Try to keep the person aware of the present environment Use distractions such as music, television, or objects
6. Sundowning (wandering)	Let the patient pace in a safe area but keep a close eye on him or her (interfering can cause anger and hostility)
7. Paranoia (patient feels the world is against him or her)	If the client accuses someone of stealing money, give them a small wallet with some money in it
8. Physical and Verbal Combativeness	Identify possible stress situations and avoid them Recognize when medication management is indicated
9. Refusal to Cooperate	Keep the environment as quiet and calm as possible
10. Separation Anxiety	Be sure the caregiver is familiar to the patient Keep the client in familiar surroundings
11. Restlessness and Anxiety	Offer the client something to hold, such as a doll or stuffed animal Try music therapy
12. Loss of Emotion	Try finger painting or other childhood games

REVIEW QUESTIONS

1. One out of every _____ Americans will be affected by Alzheimer's disease.
2. Two forms of AD are _____ and _____.
3. _____ is the term used to describe the nighttime wandering of an AD client.
4. Which of the following is not a characteristic of Stage II AD?
    a. driving problems
    b. slow walk
    c. paranoia and hostility
    d. occasional incontinence

5. Which of the following is not usually a characteristic of Stage III AD?
    a. muteness
    b. screaming
    c. wandering or sundowning
    d. dependence
6. True or False? In Stage III AD clients are often bedridden.
7. True or False? The cause of AD is a virus.
8. True or False? An objective for HCAs working with clients with AD is to promote the client's dignity.
9. Unscramble the following important key term from the chapter: wnndosugni _____

CHAPTER 4

HCA Roles and Functions

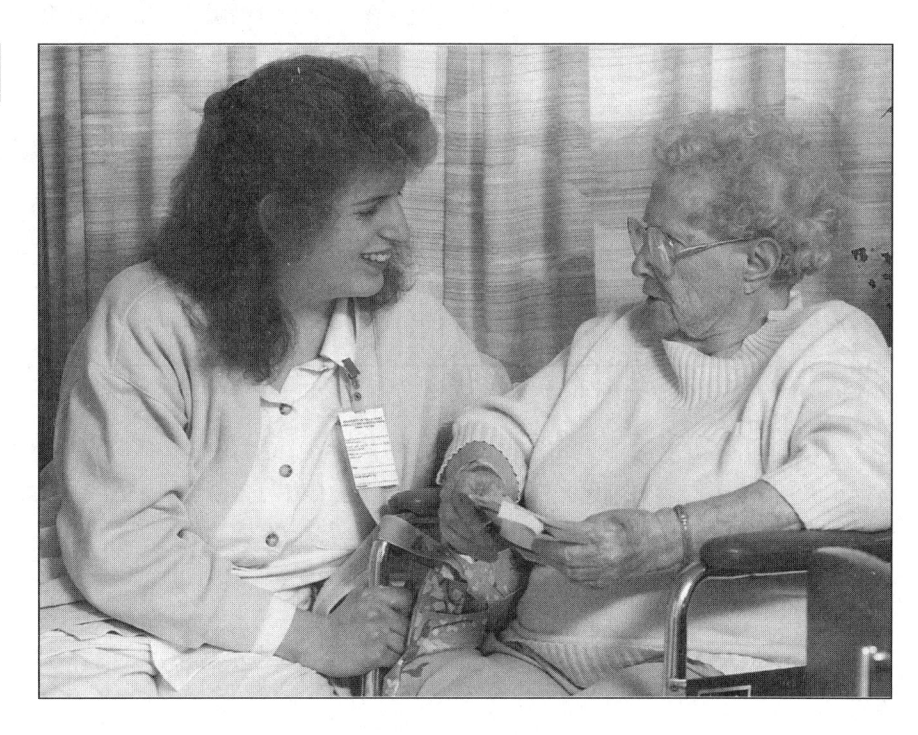

OBJECTIVES

Upon reading this chapter and completing the review questions, the home care aide should be able to:

1. Describe four primary areas of observation in judging the progression of AD.
2. List basic daily observations.
3. Be familiar with appropriate ways to report to the supervisor.
4. Describe the paperwork commonly used in documentation.
5. Recognize the rules for documentation, both general and specific, for clients with AD.
6. Be familiar with the HCA care plan, especially the activities and approaches for caring for clients with AD.

KEY TERMS

agitated
deteriorates
documentation
HCA care plan

impulsive
indicators
visit form

INTRODUCTION

The management of the client with AD is complex and involves a team of trained and untrained persons. This course prepares the HCA to assist the case manager in caring for the client with AD. The case manager is most likely the nurse assigned to the case. The care of these clients extends over a long period of time and it is important that management focus on providing long-term, cost-effective, quality care to the client with AD.

OBSERVATION AND REPORTING

When caring for a client with AD, health caregivers need to recognize **indicators** of the progression of the disease. The four primary areas of observation when judging the progression of the disease are listed below:

1. **Impulsive** Behaviors
   - does the client say inappropriate things that he or she would never had said before, or does the client use profanity?
   - does the client show a lack of understanding of his or her own safety?
2. Spatial Perception
   - does the client have depth perception, or does he or she misinterpret images on television, figures on the wall, shadows, reflections, floor patterns, or mirrors?
   - can the client eat from a plate?
3. Judgment
   - is the client able to dress himself or herself appropriately?
   - does the client recognize unsafe situations?
   - does the client ask for help when he or she needs it?
4. Insight
   - does the client realize his or her memory is inaccurate?
   - does the client voluntarily give up unsafe activities such as driving or taking his or her own medications?

The client with AD **deteriorates** in a slow, progressive manner. It is important that everyone involved be aware of the client's mental and physical status as well as his or her activity levels on a daily basis. The HCA will be with the client for extended periods of time (up to twenty-four hours) and is in a position to utilize observation and reporting as a good communication tool. It is also important that any changes in the client's status be reported to the supervisor quickly so that the team can respond appropriately. Figure 4–1 shows the communication process between the client and the HCA along with other members of the health care team.

---

indicators signs that point to specific disorders

impulsiveness an arousing of the mind to take unpremeditated action

deteriorte to make or become worse in quality or condition

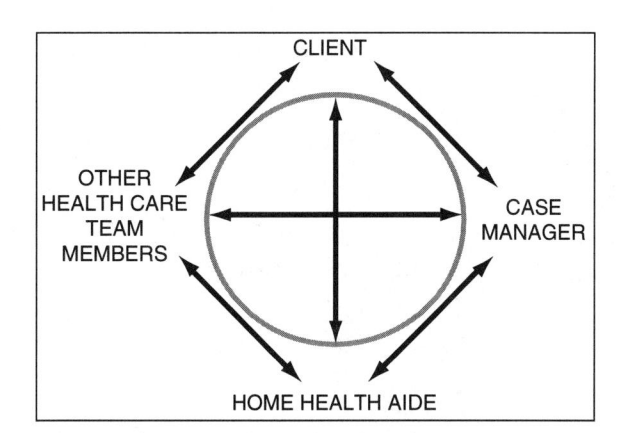

Figure 4–1 The HCA needs to interact with all members of the health care team and is an important member of the team.

The HCA should observe the home environment for safety factors as well as for adequate nutrition and proper home maintenance. The home should be maintained in an orderly, healthy, and clean manner. If the family is extremely busy, housekeeping tasks might fall to outside help. It is important that the environment be clean and free from risk of infection. It is especially important that the kitchen and food handling and storage be maintained in a sanitary manner. The client's bedroom and bathroom should be kept clean and floors uncluttered. The HCA who sees the home in need of additional outside help should report to the supervisor so that problems can be addressed.

The basic observations that should be recorded every day, or every time the HCA is in the home, and reported to the supervisor (if appropriate) include the following:

- elevated temperature
- mood changes
- decrease or increase in food or fluid intake
- changes in the skin such as bruises, bumps, sores, rashes, or skin breakdown
- changes in walking patterns such as unsteadiness, balance problems, or agitation
- swelling of joints
- deformity
- loss of function
- injury to a limb
- eye changes such as sensitivity to light, discharge from the eyes, or a fixed stare
- swelling in the ankles, feet, buttocks, or face
- changes in respiration such as shortness of breath, noisy breathing, or coughing
- changes in the mouth or tongue such as sores or swelling
- complaints of pain

- excessive flatus or abdominal distention
- poor appetite
- difficulty eating
- diarrhea or constipation
- urinary problems such as painful urination or abnormal characteristics of urine
- incontinence
- falls

Helpful Hints: Clients with AD may change their behavior from day to day; therefore, the HCA must document these behaviors accurately on each visit.

When calling the supervisor, it is important to be prepared with the answers to the following questions:

1. What is the specific observation and how is it different from the client's normal pattern?
2. When was the change observed? By whom?
3. How severe is the problem?
4. What is the client's response to the problem?
5. What are the vital signs?
6. Has any action been taken to solve the problem?

HCAs should observe clients each time they are with them, but especially when they are giving personal care. This is an excellent time to observe the client's body for any signs of elder abuse or skin breakdown.

DOCUMENTATION

documentation a written account of actions and observations

visit form a guide for the HCA to document routine and specific duties including treatments, procedueres, and observations (objective, accurate, and legible recording is necessary)

Documentation is the written account of activities, procedures, and observations in the client's home. The client's record, or chart, contain documentation from all members of the home care team. The daily **visit form** usually has space for documenting each and every treatment, procedure, and observation. The client's record is a legal document; therefore, objective, accurate, and legible recording is important. The following are guidelines for documentation:

1. The client record is written evidence of the care given, the client's response, and the outcome of the care.
2. The client's record reflects changes in orders so that all members of the health care team can keep current on new developments.
3. The client's record is a communication tool upon which the plan for care is based.
4. The client's record is a written document required by insurance companies and regulatory agencies.
5. The client's record may be used in court to prove that care was or was not given and observations documented.

Table 4–1 shows examples of documentation for the HCA.

Table 4–1 Examples of Documenting Client Behaviors

Client Actions	Observations
agitating other clients	3:00 AM—out of bed, talking to self and sounds loud and angry
confused	2:10 AM—the client states over and over that he or she wants to see his or her mother
disoriented	1:00 AM—states "I want to go to church today because it is Sunday."
combative	9:30 PM—hit nursing assistant 2X on upper arm with fist when nursing assistant attempted to change incontinent pad.
uncooperative	1:00 PM—refused to get up from chair when nursing assistant tried to take to bathroom.
verbally abusive	2:20 PM—called wife a "stupid, ignorant idiot."
physically abusive	10:00 AM—scratched nursing assistant on face when bed was being changed.

Every agency has its own records and forms. Employees should receive an orientation as to the paperwork used in their agency and become familiar with the documentation policies of their employer. Some of the forms the HCA might be required to fill out include:

- ADL sheets (see Figure 4–2)
- daily visit forms
- graph sheets for TPRs
- **HCA care plan**
- client information sheet
- team conference sheet

HCA care plan a plan developed by the nurse or supervisor as a guide to the care offered, and which contains expected client goals and outcomes

HCAs spend more time with the client than any other members of the health care team. They should be the ones to observe the client for changes in condition, especially if the changes are negative. They are the eyes and ears of the nurse and it is their responsibility to observe, document, and report everything.

Signs are changes seen, heard, felt, or smelled. Symptoms are those complaints the clients tell about and describe. HCAs should report changes in signs and symptoms to their supervisor. When reporting to the supervisor, the HCA must also document the information in written form on the client's record and include the name and title of the person to whom they verbally reported.

CHAPTER 4

Figure 4–2 Example of documenting client behaviors.

Name Cedrone, Paul						Room 311		
Activities of Daily Living								
DATE	7/14							
I. DIET: 11-7	7-3	3-11	11-7	7-3	3-11	11-7	7-3	3-11
A. MEALS-AMT. EATEN	all	all						
B. NOURISHMENTS								
II. PERSONAL HYGIENE								
A. Complete bath								
B. Assist								
C. Self	✓							
D. Shower/tub bath								
E. Mouth care	X2							
F. Peri care								
G. Back care								
III. ACTIVITY								
A. Bed rest	✓							
B. Dangle								
C. C&B								
D. BRP								
E. Ambulate								
F. ROM								
IV. Elimination								
A. Bowels	X1							
1. Amount	small							
2. Consistency	liq.							
3. Enema and results								
4. Incontinent								
B. Bladder								
1. Voided	X3							
2. Catheterized								
3. Catheter care								
4. Incontinent								
V. TREATMENTS								
1. Leg exercised TCDB								
2. Antiembol. stockings - removed and replaced								
3. Dressing changes								
4. Irrigations								
5. Soaks - hot packs, cold packs								
VI. SPECIMENS (Specify)								
VII. DIAGNOSTIC TESTS								
VIII. OTHER	stool gu neg ↑↓							
IX. SIDE RAILS UP								
X. SLEEP (naps, well, poorly)	naps							
XI. Signature	S. Lopez N.A.							

There are some general rules basic to all documentation. They include the following:

1. Recording should be descriptive, with a note about each complaint or problem.
2. Use descriptive words rather than general terms such as "normal" or "good."
3. Writing should be neat and legible.
4. Recording should be done in black ink.
5. Recording should begin with the date and time and end with a signature and title.
6. Recording should have the time a change was noted. In long-term cases, a note should be recorded at least every two hours.
7. When quoting the client's symptoms, use quotation marks.

8. All attempts to report to the supervisor should be carefully documented. If a message is left, write on the record with whom you spoke, the date, and the time.
9. Errors should not be erased, but a line drawn through the wrong entry, "mistaken entry" written, and your initials placed next to it.
10. Abbreviations used should only be those accepted by the agency.
11. If a new page is added, the client's name must appear on each page, and the time, date, and signature written again.

Because the care of the client with AD is complicated, communication among all health caregivers is vital. Documentation is of primary importance for this communication. The insurance company (such as Medicare) will be looking for validation of personal care given and the HCA's home maintenance and nutritional tasks. Specific documentation for the client with AD includes:

- signs of abuse
- changes in the client's physical or mental status
- personality changes such as increased hostilities
- behavioral changes such as self-destructive or combative behavior toward the caregivers
- positive care techniques that are particularly successful
- family problems
- incidents that occurred such as the client wandering away from the home
- fluid intake and output
- signs of infection
- problems in cooperation between the family and HCA
- signs that a social worker might be indicated
- spiritual support needed for the family or client
- daily logging of elimination patterns
- incontinence
- response to outside support groups
- signs of malnutrition
- inability of the client to care for himself or herself
- denture changes indicating a need for a dentist
- stress levels of the caregiver
- signs of skin breakdown

The following is an example of a case scenario, followed by the HCA's written observations.

agitated excitied; to move with an irregular or rapid motion

Mrs. R is a client with moderately severe AD and a history of symptoms for the past eight years. Her ability to assist with her own care has deteriorated rapidly in the last six months. The HCA has been instructed to observe the client and the home for signs of the inability of the client to remain in her environment or the possible need for outside care. At 10:00 AM, the HCA arrives at the home and finds the client in bed with apparently old, incontinent feces still on her body. The client has a fixed stare and appears to be very angry and **agitated**. The client's daughter is crying and states, "I don't think I can do this any more. I'm so tired. I didn't get any sleep until 5 o'clock this morning. My mother yelled all night."

Documentation of this case should read as follows:

10:15 AM—Arrived to find client in bed, agitated, and with incontinent sheets. Took TPRs and blood pressure: 98–100–28–180/90. Personal care given. Complete bed bath. Small red blister noted on the client's sacral area. Back rub and position change provided. Client's skin is very dry and no observable fluids at the bedside. Daughter states, "My mother refuses to drink from a cup or a straw even though I've tried her favorite juice." Skin care given, including lotion to entire body area.

11:00 AM—supervisor notified of incontinence, agitation, skin condition, and daughter's mental status.

HCA CARE PLAN

The HCA care plan is an important tool in the management process. The care plan should be developed by the nurse or supervisor on the case and used by the HCA as a guide to what care is being offered and what the goals for the client are.

An example of a care plan appropriate for all types of clients is shown in Figure 4–3. The "specific treatment and instructions" section should be adapted by the nurse for the client with AD. The nurse can make the HCA care plan individualized for each client based on that client's nursing diagnoses, goals, and expected outcomes. As the client's condition improves or changes, the nurse continually updates the care plan in the "changes" section. Notice that the HCA assignment form is divided into six patient status sections to include on the client visit. These include:

Mental Status

Incontinence

Toileting

Impairments

Mobility Aids

Activities

BOSTON REGIONAL MEDICAL CENTER/HEALTH CARE AT HOME

Home Health Aide Assignment

Client Name: _____ I.D.#: _____
Address: _____ Telephone#: (____) ____ - ____
Contact Person: _____ Telephone#: (____) ____ - ____
Directions to Home: _____
Diagnosis: _____ Age: _____
Fee Source: _____
Other Disciplines Following:
____HHA   ____R.N.   ____P.T.   ____O.T.   ____S.T.   ____S.W.

Patient Status:

Mental Status:	Incontinence:	Toileting:	Impairments:	Mobility Aids:	Activities:
—Alert	—Bowel	—Bedpan	—Speech	—Cane	—Ambulatory
—Forgetful	—Bladder	—Commode	—Hearing	—Walker	—Amb w/Ass't.
—Confused		—Bathroom	—Vision	—Crutches	—Bed Bound
—Depressed		—Catheter	—Sensation	—W/C	—W/C Bound
		—Urinal	—Paralysis	—Prosthesis	
			—Contracture	—Other	
			—Amputation		
			—Decubiti		

ASSIGNMENT: Check or circle appropriate items. Indicate frequency of assignment (eg: pm; 1 x wk; etc.)

PERSONAL CARE:
☐ Bath-sponge
☐ Bath-Tub/Shower
☐ Bath-Partial
☐ Hair-Shampoo/Grooming
☐ Nails and/or Shave
☐ Mouth Care
☐ Bed Making
☐ Help with Dressing
☐ Help with Toileting
☐ Transfer to Wheelchair
☐ Turn every—hours
☐ Lotion/Massage
☐
☐

NUTRITION:
☐ Special Diet
☐ Meal Preparation
☐ Encourage Fluids
☐ Feeding/Serving

HOUSEHOLD: Marketing
☐ Laundry
☐ Care of Bedroom
☐ Care of Kitchen
☐ Care of Bathroom
☐ Care of Living Room
☐ Linen Change
☐ Light Housework
☐

SPECIAL SERVICES:
☐ Exercise if requested by PT/RN
☐ Ambulation-Walker, etc.
☐ Special Skin Care
☐ Weigh Patient
☐ Measure intake/output
☐ Check bowel elimination
☐ Assist with Medication
☐ Accompany to M.D.
☐ Pulse, Respiration and B.P.
☐ Temperature-Oral/Axillary
☐ Dressing Change/Wound Care
☐ Ostomy Care
☐ Catheter Care/Empty Drainage Bag
☐

BP:_____ Pulse: _____
Other:_____

ADDITIONAL INSTRUCTIONS/SAFETY PRECAUTIONS:
_____
_____
_____
_____
_____

Signature of Nurse/Therapist: _____ Date: _____
Freq/Visits: _____ Preference of Days: _____ Time: ____ AM ____ PM
Case Manager: _____ Primary HHA: _____ Date: _____
Signature of Assigned Personnel: _____

ASSIGNMENT REVIEW:
Date: _____ Initials: _____ Date: _____ Initials: _____
Date: _____ Initials: _____ Date: _____ Initials: _____
Date: _____ Initials: _____ Date: _____ Initials: _____

EMERGENCY NUMBERS:
Distribution: Yellow   —   Chart
                Pink   —   HHA
                Green   —   Patient's Home

Figure 4–3 These are the assigned duties of the home health aide. (Courtesy Boston Regional Medical Center/ Health Care at Home, Stoneham, MA)

The other three main sections to address are personal care, nutrition, and special services.

Some activities that could be added to the general HCA care plan specific to Alzheimer's include:

- observation of mental status of the family and the client
- vital signs
- assistance with ADLs
- understanding the progression of the disease
- weight loss
- special mouth care
- elimination patterns
- safety measures
- orientation
- catheter care
- daily exercises
- assistive devices
- repositioning of the client
- skin care
- level of mobility

HCA VISIT FORM

Figure 4–4 is an example of a visit form for the HCA caring for the client with AD. The form was developed to guide the HCA through the procedures that are to be done at each visit. There are observation requirements for each visit and specific procedures for clients with AD that are performed on some clients but not on others. For these reasons, the visit form is divided into a section of routine tasks that should be done on every visit, and a section showing specific duties which the nurse will instruct the HCA to perform for that specific client. The HCA daily visit form is the most important communication tool between the HCA and the nurse and it is important that the HCA make it a part of his or her routine.

Helpful Hints: The nurse assigned to the case reads the HCA's notes for information concerning the client's progress and it is important that the HCA document accurately and legibly at all times.

HOME CARE AIDE VISIT FORM FOR ALZHEIMER'S DISEASE				
Patient's Name:	No:	Diagnosis:		Insulin Therapy:
Diet	Nurse:		Date Begin Plan:	Date Discharge:
Routine Care:	Date:	Documentation:		Sign:

☐ Observe Skin
    ☐ Reddened areas
    ☐ Positioning for pressure points
    ☐ Ulcerations/blisters
    ☐ Wound
☐ Observe/assist Elimination
    ☐ Incontinent
        ☐ Bowel
        ☐ Bladder
    ☐ Constipation
    ☐ Fecal impaction
    ☐ Diarrhea
    ☐ Elimination care
        ☐ Catheter
        ☐ Depends®
    ☐ Bathroom training
        ☐ Diary
        ☐ Coping practices
        ☐ Safety devices
        ☐ Portable commode
☐ Observe/assist Nutrition
    ☐ Adequate fluid intake and output
    ☐ Fiber diet for bowel training
    ☐ Encourage/restrict fluids for bladder training
    ☐ Special diet high calorie/soft
    ☐ Needs feeding assistance
    ☐ Feeds Self
    ☐ Prepares own foods
    ☐ Caregiver prepares foods
☐ Observe/assist Home Maintenance
    ☐ Self care
    ☐ Patient Independent (10–100%) _____
    ☐ Patient needs assistance
    ☐ Patient totally dependent
☐ Observe/assist Activity/Ambulation
    ☐ PT ☐ OT ☐ ST
    ☐ Patient disabled (10–100%) _____
    ☐ Requires assistance
    ☐ Assisting devices
    ☐ Environment healthy and clean
    ☐ Sundowning (freq. per week _____)
☐ Observe Safety
    ☐ Visual problems
    ☐ Hearing problems
    ☐ Unsteady, requires assistance
    ☐ Environment safe
        ☐ Precautions _____
    ☐ Patient understands safety measures
        ☐ (10–100%) _____
☐ Observe/assist Personal Care
    ☐ Bathing
        ☐ Self   ☐ Partial assist
        ☐ Shower with assistance
        ☐ Complete care
    ☐ Oral hygiene   ☐ Self   ☐ Assist
    ☐ Hair care
    ☐ Shave
    ☐ Nail care
☐ Observe Mental Status
    ☐ Confusion
    ☐ Oriented
    ☐ Forgetfulness
    ☐ Agitation
    ☐ Anxiety
    ☐ Fearful
    ☐ Reality orientation frequency_____
☐ Observe Communication
    ☐ Coherent
    ☐ Speaks clearly
    ☐ Verbal (10–100%) _____				

Figure 4–4 AD Visit Form (Courtesy of Health Education, Inc., Ft Lauderdale, FL)

REVIEW QUESTIONS

1. Four primary areas of observation of the client with AD for judging the progress of the disease are:

   a.

   b.

   c.

   d.

2. The best time to observe the client's skin is _____
3. _____ is the written account of activities, procedures, and observations.
4. The _____ develops the HCA care plan.
5. Which of the following is/are not included in the HCA care plan?

   a. nutrition and mental status

   b. safety and elimination

   c. physical therapy and occupational therapy

   d. activity and personal care

6. Which are specific activities to add to the general HCA care plan for caring for the client with AD?

   a. progression of disease

   b. weight loss

   c. mental status of family

   d. all of the above

7. Which of the following is not usually included in the information the HCA obtains when preparing to call the supervisor?

   a. where the problem is

   b. when has the client had the problem before

   c. The HCA's feeling

   d. client's description of the pain

8. True or False? It is important that health caregivers be aware of the AD client's mental status on a daily basis.
9. True or False? Safety factors are the responsibility of the family and the physical therapist.
10. True or False? It is important to prepare for calls to the supervisor.
11. True or False? Only the HCA records and documents information on the client's record.

Indicate with a "yes" or "no" whether each term is appropriate for proper documentation.

12. descriptive words and phrases
13. general words and phrases
14. blue ink
15. signature
16. legible handwriting

17. information about who and when
18. changes
19. family problems.
20. Unscramble the following important key term from the chapter: mtocuedntonai
    _____

CHAPTER 5

Care of the Client with Alzheimer's Disease

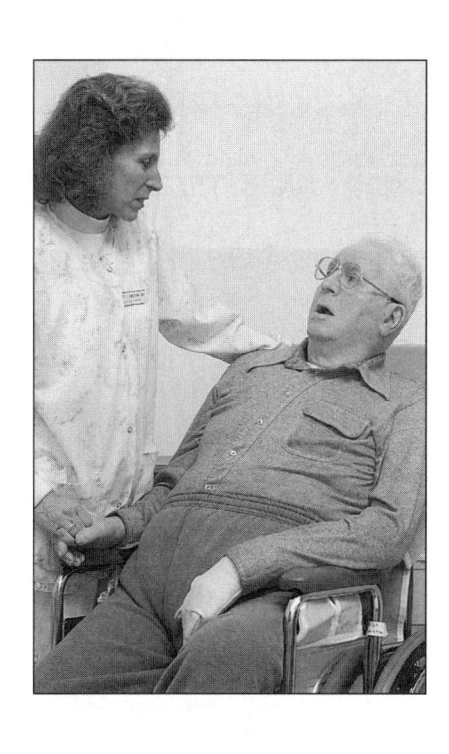

OBJECTIVES

appropriate response a response that is suitable for a particular situation

Upon reading this chapter and completing the review questions, the home care aide should be able to:

1. Describe basic techniques for caring for clients with Alzheimer's disease.
2. Be familiar with problem behaviors of the client with Alzheimer's disease and **appropriate responses**.
3. Define problem areas in communication with clients with Alzheimer's disease and guidelines for action and appropriate responses.
4. Define incontinence and the effects on the client with Alzheimer's disease, health problems, and caregiving guidelines.
5. Define sundowning and coping strategies.
6. Describe personal hygiene and approaches in the care of the client with Alzheimer's disease.
7. Recognize the importance of good nutrition as it applies to the client with ALzheimer's disease.

KEY TERMS

appropriate responses
delusions
distraction
hallucinates
techniques
voice intonation

INTRODUCTION

technique systematic approach or procedure used to accomplish a task

There are five main areas of concern or caring challenges when considering the care of the client with AD. These include communication, incontinence, sundowning, personal hygiene, and nutrition. Because caring for the client with AD is difficult and often confusing, the specialized HCA develops particular **techniques** for caring for these persons.

COMMUNICATION

Communicating with any elderly client can be a challenge for the HCA. The client with AD, however, may not be able to understand what others are saying or not be able to make himself or herself understood. This creates an even greater challenge to the health caregiver or family caregiver. Some common communication problems are:

- the client might substitute a word that sounds similar to the word he or she cannot remember
- the client might try to describe thoughts or objects
- the client might invent new words to describe thoughts or objects
- the client might use words over and over (this includes swearing or making offensive remarks)
- the client cannot verbalize long thoughts
- the client might become angry when verbalizing is difficult
- the client might become frustrated and fearful when he or she is having problems communicating
- the client might cry and become depressed if the person with whom he or she is trying to communicate becomes frustrated (this increases the response in the client)

It is important to discuss some reactions health caregivers have to certain communication behaviors. In the early stages of AD, communication can be improved by the use of signs and labels which are reassuring to the client. As the disease progresses, however, the client might be unable to speak, and nonverbal communication such as touch or laughter can be helpful. The person with AD responds more to touch than to words. Holding his or her hand or putting your arm around the shoulder with a slow and gentle stroking motion is calming for the client. Some individuals do not like to be touched, however, and the HCA

CARE OF THE CLIENT WITH ALZHEIMER'S DISEASE 41

should respect this response. The following is a list of tips for communicating with the client with AD:

1. Make sure you have the client's attention before you begin to speak. Make sure that he or she can see and hear you and knows that you are speaking to him or her.
2. Face the client when you speak and speak slowly and clearly.
3. Do not talk too much and give only one instruction at a time.
4. Speak in positives instead of negatives. The client will respond better to "Come with me," than to "Come away from there!"
5. Listen carefully to what the client is saying: it might be important.
6. Respond to the client' feelings, not just his or her words.
7. Focus on validation, not on reality orientation.
8. Be aware of body language.
9. If the client is frustrated because he or she is unable to make you understand, reassure him or her that you still care about what the client feels: "I'm sorry I can't understand what you are saying. Why don't you wait a while and try to tell me later?" Move on to another activity.
10. Never ask, "Do you remember . . . ?" Instead, tell the client what you want him or her to remember: "We went to your doctor's office on Tuesday, and he said that you need to drink more water."

Facial expressions, such as a smile, shows that the HCA is paying attention. The client with AD also communicates with non-verbal gestures and facial expressions and these should be considered forms of communication. Figure 5–1 shows an HCA communicating with a client.

Helpful Hints: Clients with AD are sensitive to facial expressions of disgust or anger. The HCA must be careful to avoid making these facial expressions.

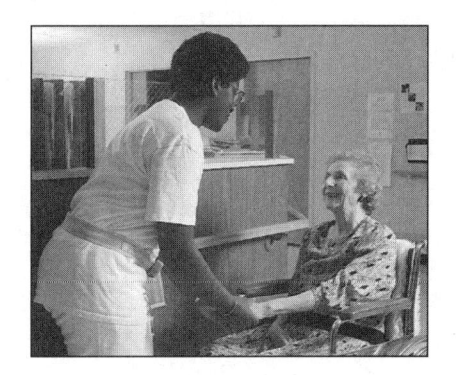

Figure 5–1 The HCA is showing affection by using touch to reassure the AD client.

Any communication that shows affection and patience is excellent in the HCA's approach to these clients. Some suggestions for assisting the client to communicate his or her message are:

- Be calm and supportive. The HCA should maintain eye contact and use appropriate touch to reassure the client that he or she is listening.
- Show interest in what the client is saying with facial gestures of concern and interest.
- Pay attention to his or her voice and gestures for clues to what the client is feeling. Many times, this is more important than what the client is trying to say.
- If the HCA does not understand the verbal message, acknowledge that and ask the client to point or gesture.
- If the client cannot find a word, the HCA can lower the frustration level by offering a guess.
- If the client uses the wrong word and the HCA knows what he or she wants to say, supply the correct word. If, however, this practice upsets the client, do not repeat it.
- If the client gets upset because he or she is unable to give a verbal explanation, do not encourage the client to attempt more conversation. Offer comfort and reassurance instead.

Nine guidelines for the HCA to consider when developing a course of action for communication with the client with AD are:

1. Determine if a hearing problem exists.
2. Never talk about the client as if he or she is not there.
3. Use signs or written messages.
4. Use nonverbal communication.
5. Be calm and supportive.
6. Give undivided attention to the client
7. Encourage pointing and gesturing.
8. Offer a guess.
9. Use humor when possible.

The Alzheimer's Association has done a great deal of research in developing techniques to assist caregivers to communicate with the client with AD. The following are adapted from the Alzheimer's Association's list for "Helping the Person Understand What You are Saying:"

- Approach the client from the front, but be aware that some persons feel more comfortable by keeping a handshake distance away.
- Keep confusion and noise to a minimum and do not startle the client.

- Begin each conversation by identifying yourself and addressing the client to orient him or her and to get his or her attention.
- Speak slowly and distinctly. Use a lower pitched voice to convey a sense of calm. This also enables the hearing impaired person to hear better.
- Pay attention to the tone of voice used. Tone is as important as the words spoken because the client can sense emotion and is sensitive to nonverbal messages.
- Use short, simple, familiar words and sentences. Speak slowly, and do not expect a quick response.
- Explain actions and break tasks and instructions into clear, simple steps. Give one step at a time.
- Ask one question or offer one idea at a time and give the client time to respond. Rushing him or her increases confusion.
- Repeat questions or information using the same phrasing and words as before.
- Touch an arm or shoulder to get the client's attention and maintain eye contact.
- Talk in positive terms. Limit the use of the word "don't" and avoid giving harsh and direct orders. Use direct statements such as "It is time to get dressed now."
- Avoid expressions that the client may take too literally such as "hop into bed."
- Demonstrate a request by drawing, pointing at, or touching things.
- Use names when referring to other individuals instead of using "her" or "she."
- Treat the client with dignity and respect; remember that he or she is an adult. Do not "talk down" to the client simply because you are using simple words or sentences.
- Do not use pet name such as "honey"; they can sound condescending.
- Ignore harmless hallucinations or **delusions**. Confronting the client can make the situation worse. Respond with reassurance and distract the client toward another activity.
- Try to communicate the same message a few minutes later if the client appears to not be paying attention.
- Use nonverbal communication such as a smile or a hug to reinforce verbal communication. Remember that facial expressions are as important as words.

delusion a false belief despite acceptable facts to the contrary

Helpful Hints: If the HCA feels stressed or unable to cope with caring for a client with AD, he or she should talk to the supervisor about a change of assignment.

When caring for these difficult clients, it is important that the HCA be empowered to take care of himself or herself. It is common for nurses and HCAs to want to please the family and the client but being assertive enough to say "no" with poise and confidence is important when request for the HCA's time and energy are not realistic. Keep in mind that by saying "no" to a situation that is not appropriate to your role and functions, you are not rejecting the person making the request, but simply saying "no" to the request itself. An appropriate response would be, "No, that is not appropriate under my assignment at this time."

There will be many opportunities for HCAs to be the motivating forces in the care of the client with AD at home. Their communication skills will grow in a positive way and the rewards will be many.

The following are typical communication problems with dementia clients and their appropriate responses:

Communication Problem	Appropriate Response
Forgets what was said	Repeat using same words or phrases
Substitutes words	Suggest word, but if it upsets the client, use a smile and touch to show caring
Questions over and over	Answer each time
Cannot verbalize	Encourage gestures
Lives in past	Encourage reminiscing
Hallucinates	Ignore or use distractions; validate feelings
Confusion about tasks	Break into simple steps
Repeats	Accept this as part of the disease process
Afraid of you	Move and speak slowly; use simply sentences and give nonverbal messages of caring
Verbally abusive	Ignore
Sad or crying	Listen; try distraction and touch, slowly

hallucinates an illusion of something that does not exist

INCONTINENCE

Incontinence is the loss of control of urination and/or bowel elimination. As with any chronic problem of incontinence, the HCA will be involved with the problems resulting from this loss of body function. If the client is in the early stages of AD, accidents usually occur only once or twice a week. Figure 5–2 is an illustrative guide to help the HCA understand and remember the causes of incontinence.

CARE OF THE CLIENT WITH ALZHEIMER'S DISEASE 45

ABC of Incontinence

Helen Smith, an EN at Hither Green Hospital, has devised an illustrative guide to help nurses during their geriatric experience to understand and remember the causes of incontinence.

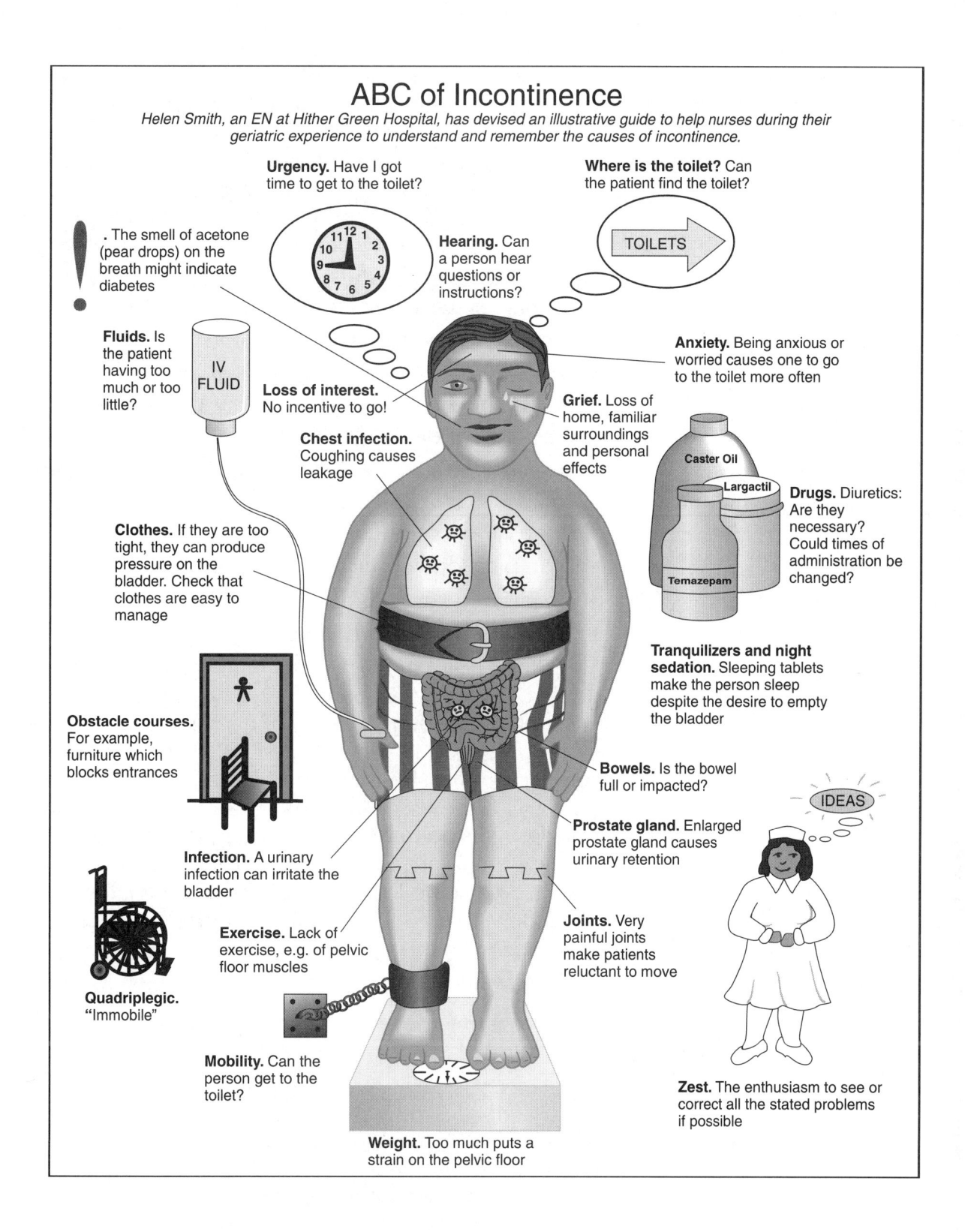

Urgency. Have I got time to get to the toilet?

Where is the toilet? Can the patient find the toilet?

. The smell of acetone (pear drops) on the breath might indicate diabetes

Hearing. Can a person hear questions or instructions?

Fluids. Is the patient having too much or too little?

Loss of interest. No incentive to go!

Anxiety. Being anxious or worried causes one to go to the toilet more often

Grief. Loss of home, familiar surroundings and personal effects

Chest infection. Coughing causes leakage

Drugs. Diuretics: Are they necessary? Could times of administration be changed?

Clothes. If they are too tight, they can produce pressure on the bladder. Check that clothes are easy to manage

Tranquilizers and night sedation. Sleeping tablets make the person sleep despite the desire to empty the bladder

Obstacle courses. For example, furniture which blocks entrances

Bowels. Is the bowel full or impacted?

Prostate gland. Enlarged prostate gland causes urinary retention

Infection. A urinary infection can irritate the bladder

Joints. Very painful joints make patients reluctant to move

Quadriplegic. "Immobile"

Exercise. Lack of exercise, e.g. of pelvic floor muscles

Mobility. Can the person get to the toilet?

Zest. The enthusiasm to see or correct all the stated problems if possible

Weight. Too much puts a strain on the pelvic floor

Figure 5–2 An illustrative guide to help understand and remember the causes of incontinence. Reproduced by kind permission of *Nursing Times* where this was first published on November 13, 1985.

Incontinence in the client with AD begins in Stage II of the illness and progresses into Stage III with a gradual decline in the client's ability to control the bowel and bladder. In Stage II and early in Stage III, there is a possibility of approaching the problem of incontinence through bowel and bladder training. The procedures for bowel and bladder training are given in Chapter 6. Incontinence may be caused by any of the following factors:

- arteriosclerosis of the blood vessels that supply blood to the urinary system or sphincter muscles
- inability to get to the toilet in time
- decreased muscle tone because of age
- a loss of concentration which regulates and controls the bowels and bladder in the client with AD

Health problems associated with urinary incontinence include:

- inability to measure the client's fluid output
- skin breakdown which leads to decubitus ulcers
- inability to collect urine specimens
- personal hygiene problems

For the client in Stage II AD who is incontinent once or twice a week, the use of Depends® or other adult protection products is helpful (see Figure 5–3). The disposable briefs must be changed promptly when soiled or they defeat the purpose of preventing skin breakdown. Clients with AD who are out of touch with their surroundings will not be aware that the brief is soiled, so it is up to the caregiver to check it frequently.

Basic skin care is essential in caring for the elderly but becomes even more important when caring for the client with AD. The following are some guidelines for basic skin care:

- protect the client from scratches or skin injuries which can lead to infection

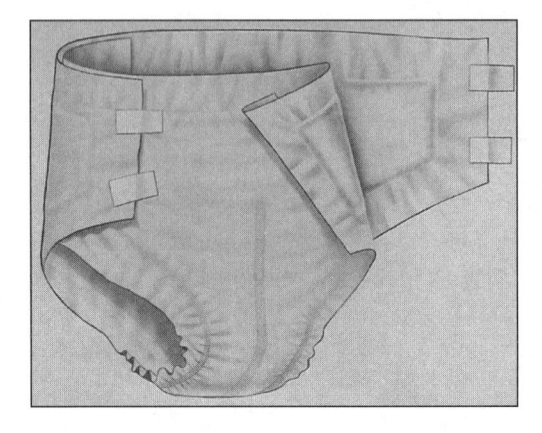

Figure 5–3 This disposable brief is used for a client who is incontinent.

- protect the client from exposure to the sun or wind
- keep the client's body as clean and dry as possible and use mild soap and rinse well (do not use bath salts because they tend to dry the skin)
- change the bed and wash bed linens as often as necessary to keep the incontinent client dry
- never use rubber pants because they are irritating to the skin. Use a bed protector (disposable, if available) and make sure its plastic side never touches the client's skin
- always discuss the type of disposable product that is best suited for the client with the supervisor
- use lotion on the skin to protect the area from bodily discharges and drainage (if using powder or corn starch, use only small amounts and wash it off at bath time)
- the client's position should be changed at least every two hours
- the family should follow the schedule when caring for the client
- never slide the client on the bed to prevent friction between the skin and the sheet (sliding causes shearing of the skin)
- never leave the client on a bedpan longer than necessary and be certain urine does not remain on the skin (powdering the bedpan helps minimize friction)
- all linen should be dry and free of wrinkles and the bed free from crumbs
- check clients with catheters frequently to ensure that the catheter is flowing freely and is not caught underneath the client
- discuss with the supervisor what cream is best to use if the client's skin is dry
- never rub the skin hard; use a lotion and rub in a circular motion to stimulate blood circulation
- avoid pressure on any bony parts of the body
- provide good nutrition and adequate fluid intake

The following are some guidelines for coping with incontinence in the AD client:

1. Keep a notebook and list the time and amount of each urination. This helps to plan when to take the client to the bathroom. For example, if the client is usually continent after four hours, the HCA should take him or her to the bathroom every three hours.
2. Sometimes incontinence in the client with AD is caused by that person's inability to find the bathroom. In this situation, the

Helpful Hints: Applying lotion and performing skin care procedures should be part of every client's personal care routine and done on every visit.

Helpful Hints: Clients in Stage III AD are likely to have urinary catheters.

HCA should put something on the bathroom door that makes it stand out such as a bright color or a picture of a toilet.
3. Make sure the client with AD is dressed in clothing that can easily be undone such as jogging pants with an elastic waist.
4. Praise success and ignore inappropriate behavior. Never punish failure to urinate.
5. Stimulate reflexes that support voiding such as running the water faucet while the client is sitting on the toilet.
6. Allow the hyperactive client to get up and down from the toilet a few times. Show them with gestures that they are to sit on the toilet or offer a distraction such as a magazine or a doll to occupy them while they are sitting.
7. Construct a toilet stall with a safety bar similar to that on a ferris wheel which crosses the client's lap while they sit on the toilet. A broom or a mop handle can be cut to size. This bar prevents the unstable client from falling while sitting long enough to void or defecate.
8. Avoid skin burns from urine by cleaning with water immediately after urination. Castile soap also may be used.
9. Be sure that stress incontinence is not the problem. The use of medications that help the bladder to retain urine might help.

Helpful Hints: Clients with AD probably would not drink adequate amounts of liquids each day without the encouragement of the HCA and the family.

Constipation is a common problem in the elderly and is frequently seen in clients with AD who have poor nutritional intake. Drugs that cause constipation and lack of exercise are also factors.

It is best for the physician or the nurse to develop a bowel program for each client individually. For example, one client can regulate the bowels by adding prune juice to the diet. Another client may need a daily laxative and stool softener to avoid constipation. Every person has different ranges for normal bowel movements. Some persons move their bowels once a day and others two or three times a day. Constipation is the retention of fecal matter along with difficult passage of hard stools. A fecal impaction is a large amount of hard stool in the lower rectum and is a very painful condition. If this occurs, the nurse might have to remove it manually. It is very important for the HCA to keep a careful log of bowel movements or attempted bowel movements. If the client frequently experiences the feeling of needing to move the bowels but is unable to do so, constipation or an impaction could be indicated.

SUNDOWNING

Sundowning is a term used to describe the confusion that commonly occurs in clients with AD late in the day, especially after

CARE OF THE CLIENT WITH ALZHEIMER'S DISEASE 49

Helpful Hints: Clients with AD who wander should always wear identification bracelets in case they get lost.

dark. Sundowning causes great anxiety in the confused and insecure client and results in the restless wandering of many clients. It is a very dangerous condition if the client is alone outside the home. Unfortunately, sundowning has caused the death of many clients with AD as they wandered away from the home into traffic or got lost in underpopulated areas. Figure 5–4 shows a client with AD wandering away from his family.

Sundowning occurs whether the client with AD lives in familiar surroundings or in a facility, but it is worse after a move or change in routine. The cause of sundowning is unknown, but it is assumed that these persons become emotionally fatigued because of their inability to concentrate, thereby resulting in their restlessness. It is also though that darkness is frightening to the client with AD who is already disoriented. It is important that the caregivers and the family understand that the client with AD is in a state of fear. They should provide reassurance and protection and keep doors locked to protect the client.

Similar to schizophrenia, clients with AD who wander from the home may see and hear things that are not real. In addition, agitated clients have increased strength and energy. For example, an eighty-five-year-old client with AD who is agitated could have the energy of a five year old.

The following are helpful strategies for coping with sundowning in clients with AD:

1. Try to keep the client active in the morning and encourage a nap after lunch.
2. Let the client pace whenever possible. Physical restraints usually increase the client's level of anxiety.

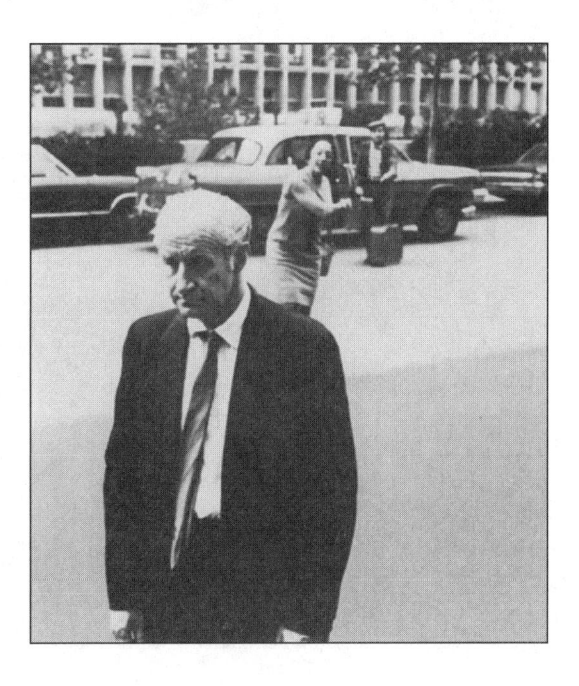

Figure 5–4 Sundowning occurs when disoriented AD clients often wander at dusk.

3. Use bean bag chairs so the client can move around without danger of falling and without physical restraints. These chairs are difficult to get out of, yet comfortable and easy to clean.
4. Give the client something to hold to keep them occupied such as stuffed animals and dolls. For clients who smoke, a lollipop can be a safe substitute when the client is in the presence of a responsible adult.
5. Eliminate bright lights and other stimuli in the evening hours.
6. Eliminate caffeine and other stimulants from the client's diet.
7. Provide a quiet and calm environment in the evening and possibly add quiet music to the surroundings to keep the client calm.

There are new mechanical devices which can protect the client, such as s tracer-type beeper so that if the client gets out of bed at night, the family will be awakened. Figure 5–5 is an example of a tracer-type bracelet. Intercoms from the client's room to the caregiver's room are also good protection. The wearing of an ID bracelet is extremely important. The bracelets should be tamper-proof and labeled with the client's name, address, and telephone number. One type of bracelet has a code on it that simply says "memory loss." Many Alzheimer's Associations have a system in which clients are enrolled. Should they wander away or become lost, the person who finds them can contact the association and the client can be returned home.

PERSONAL HYGIENE

Many elderly clients fear accidents in the tub or shower or lose interest in their appearance. The client with AD becomes a great challenge when he or she refuses to bathe, is too confused to handle the activities of daily living, or becomes hostile when a

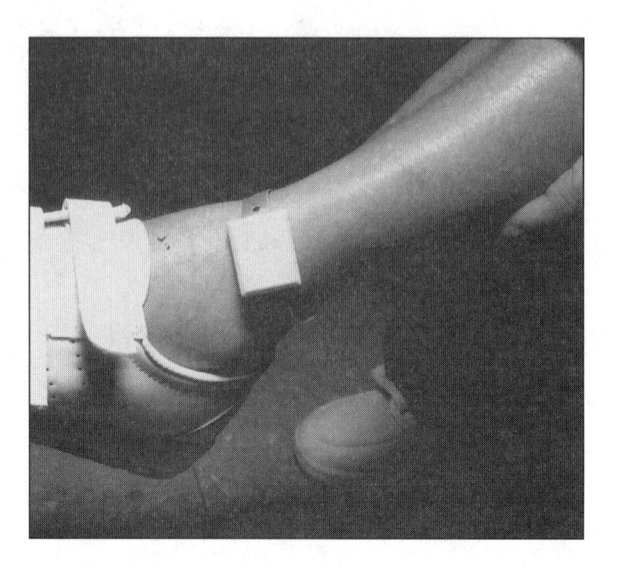

Figure 5–5 A special sensor may be attached to the leg of the wandering, disoriented client.

CARE OF THE CLIENT WITH ALZHEIMER'S DISEASE

Helpful Hints: Many clients with AD are fearful of water, baths, or showers which results in anger or combative behavior.

caregiver attempts to assist with personal hygiene. The client frequently forgets from one day to the next what activities he or she has been able to do. In some situations, it requires more than one caregiver to bathe or shower a hyperactive client with AD.

Gaining the client's trust is the first step in getting their cooperation when performing personal hygiene routines. It is important that the HCA have an excellent relationship with the client before attempting to assist with personal hygiene. Patience and gentleness are essential.

Personal hygiene for the confused and elderly client often becomes the responsibility of the caregiver, usually the HCA. Personal hygiene includes washing the client's body and grooming. It also includes the client's surroundings. The elderly are especially susceptible to infections and the home must be kept as clean as possible.

Some of the important tasks the HCA should review when preparing to assist with the personal hygiene of the client with AD include:

- infection control and standard precautions, including hand washing, gloving, and collecting specimens
- restorative care, including positioning, maintaining body alignment, transfer techniques, range of motion exercises, and assistive devices
- bathing, skin care, and perineal care
- daily care, oral hygiene, denture care, shaving, dressing, nail care, and hair care
- feeding, including intake and output recording
- toileting, including bedpans, urinals, catheters, and bowel and bladder training

Helpful Hints: Toddler toys appeal to clients with AD and are safe to use for distraction during bath time.

There are some special guidelines for bathing and personal hygiene for the client with AD. The caregiver or the HCA should avoid scheduling the bath in the late afternoon or early evening. The bath should be given when the client is the most rested and the least confused. If the client refuses the bath, the HCA should walk away and try again later. Avoid using the shower if it causes anxiety. Use techniques to help the client relax such as soft music, singing, distractions, foot massage, or a back rub. Figure 5–6 shows the HCA assisting the client with AD to take a bath. Toys in the bathtub and brightly colored soaps are helpful.

The following are guidelines for bathing the client with AD:

- try to follow as many of the client's old routines as possible
- simplify the task as much as possible
- have everything ready before starting
- talk the client through each step of the bath

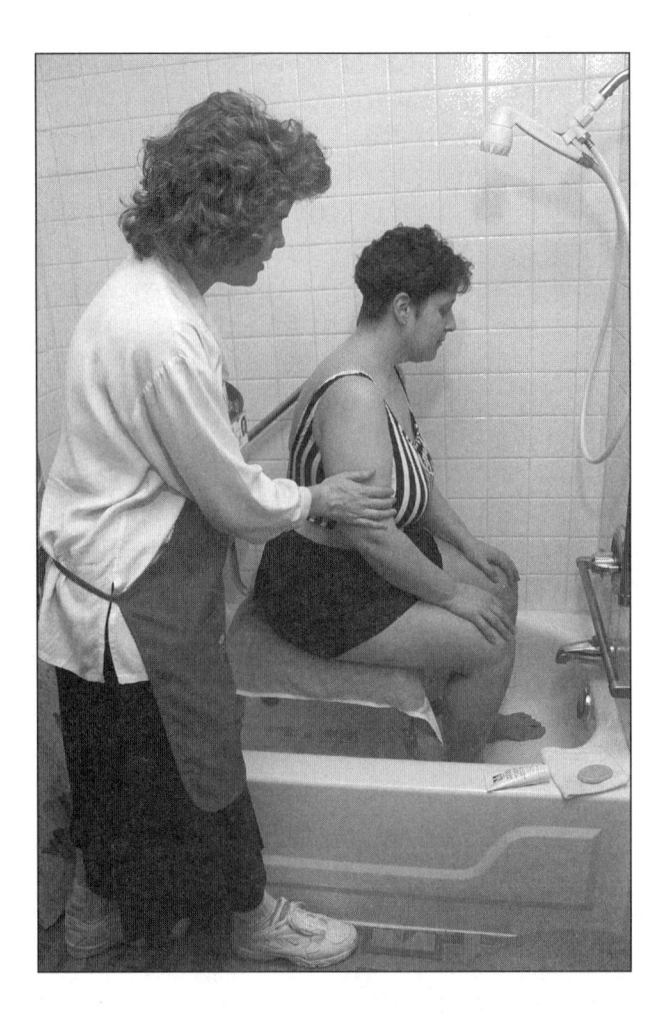

Figure 5–6 The HCA assists the client with AD with their bath and washing her back.

- do not rush or hurry the client because this creates anxiety
- do not talk about the need for the bath; talk about other things
- never force the client to bathe
- always check the temperature of the bath water
- avoid bath oils that make the tub slippery
- use proper skin care products
- use a minimal amount of water
- use safety devices such as grab bars and rubber mats
- encourage the client to do as much self-care as possible
- use the bath time as an opportunity to look for bruises, rashes, or sores
- use a belt abound the client's waist during bathing if the client seems likely to fall
- if the client refuses to get into the tub, perform a sponge bath
- try sponge baths when the client is sitting in a chair or on a bed, or even while he or she is walking around
- remove locks from the bathroom door
- do not leave hair dryers or electric razors within a client's reach

NUTRITION

Clients with AD tend to become malnourished because of their disorientation, inability to handle food, and increased restlessness which raises the body's caloric need. Providing good nutrition is an important consideration of the health caregiver, especially the HCA.

There are various factors that affect nutrition in the elderly client with or without AD. These include social factors such as:
- problems with food shopping and preparation
- lack of socialization at mealtime
- limited finances
- living alone
- lack of transportation

Psychological factors that affect nutrition in the elderly include:
- depression which causes a decrease in appetite
- loss of a spouse
- loss of self-esteem
- loss of independence

Physical factors that affect nutrition in the elderly include:
- immobility
- inability to feed oneself
- chewing difficulties

Eating factors that affect nutrition in the elderly include:
- decreased metabolism
- decreased appetite
- loss of taste and smell
- gastric problems

Disease factors that affect nutrition in the elderly include:
- medication regimen
- infection
- loss of caring about eating
- memory loss
- inability to recognize the need to eat, particularly in clients with AD.

These persons are usually dependent on someone else to provide their nutrition. The factors mentioned above are more evident in the client with AD than in other clients.

The HCA should review the daily food guide and provide the client with AD with a balanced and nutritious diet. A sample menu for a client with AD includes several servings of fruits and vegetables, several servings of milk or milk products, (cheese cubes or yogurt), two servings of meat or protein (eggs, cottage cheese, or peanut butter), decaffeinated beverages, and few fats, sweets, or alcohol. Figure 5–7 shows examples of single servings from each food group. Six to eight 8-oz. glasses of water every day prevents dehydration and promotes regular bowel function.

Recipes

Two recipes that the HCA might use for clients who refuse to eat are Feeling Good Bars and a special high-calorie milkshake.

Feeling Good Bars*
INGREDIENTS:

1 cup raisins $2/3$ cup powdered milk

1 cup water   1 teaspoon baking soda

$1/2$ cup oil   1 teaspoon ground cinnamon

1 egg $1/2$ teaspoon nutmeg

$3/4$ cup brown sugar, packed $1/4$ teaspoon ground cloves

$3/4$ cup enriched flour $1/2$ cup chopped almonds

$3/4$ cup whole wheat flour

DIRECTIONS: Combine raisins and water in saucepan and heat to boiling. Remove from heat, stir in oil, and cool to room temperature. Stir in egg and brown sugar. Sift together flour, baking

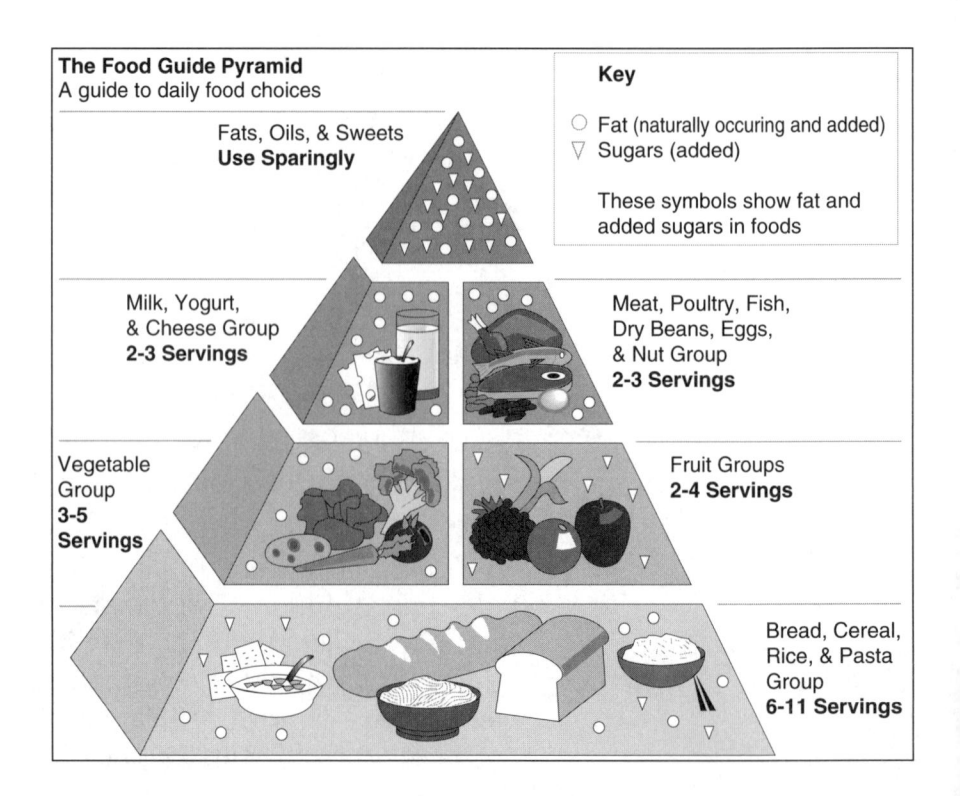

Figure 5–7 Examples of servings that form each of the food groups.

soda, and spices. Add milk. Add to raisin mixture and beat until smooth. Stir in nuts. Spread mixture in 9" x 9" baking pan coated with nonstick vegetable spray. Bake at 350° for 20 to 30 minutes or until done. YIELD: twelve 3" x 2 1/4" bars.

NUTRIENT ANALYSIS:

Calories	264
Fat	12.8 g.
Fiber	1.9 g.
Iron	1.6 g.
Calcium	137 mg.
Thiamin	0.13 mg.
Vitamin C	1 mg.
Niacin	0.9 mg.
Protein	6 g.
Carbohydrate	33.8 g.
Cholesterol	21 mg.
Sodium	77 mg.
Vitamin A	25 IU
Riboflavin	0.2 mg.
Potassium	324 mg.
Phosphorous	152 mg.

*Source: *Dietitian's Food Favorites Cookbook*. Available from the American Dietetic Association, 216 W. Jackson Boulevard, Suite 700, Chicago, IL 60606-6995.

Special High-Calorie Milkshake

INGREDIENTS:
1 8-oz. can vanilla liquid Ensure® (or Ensure HN®)
1/2 cup chocolate ice cream

DIRECTIONS:
Beat in blender or with a whisk until smooth.

NOTE: Unpasteurized or raw eggs should not be added to milkshakes or uncooked foods because of the potential for salmonella food poisoning.

Some suggestions for mealtime are:
- offer a few simple choices, one at a time
- use finger foods or small, soft pieces of food
- serve favorite foods that are nutritious
- ask the client to eat slowly and chew thoroughly
- try adaptive eating devices

> **Helpful Hints:** The HCA should be careful not to give finger foods that could result in choking the client.

- keep pet food or poisonous or dangerous items out of the client's reach
- maintain calm environment at mealtime

The dietitian can be brought into the home to help design a diet that will maintain adequate nutrition for the client with AD.

BEHAVIORS OF THE CLIENT WITH AD

The HCA should expect odd and unusual behaviors from AD clients. Some that have been recorded are:

- lighting fires if matches are around
- taking off clothes (at inappropriate times)
- accusing others of stealing
- sexual gestures
- showing anger toward the caregiver
- inappropriate laughter
- throwing food
- playing with feces

The Alzheimer's Association suggests that caregivers and others have AD clients participate in the following activities to retain and protect former behaviors:

1. To preserve the client's remote memory:
   - review their lives
   - look at old photographs, both personal and historical
   - discuss familiar topics such as crafts, sports, and the like
   - play memory games such as simple card games
   - play word games developed for children under the age of ten.
2. To preserve the client's motor function:
   - exercise and take walks
   - dance
   - play tossing games such as bean bags or play with a ball
3. Engage client in repetitive, rhythmic behaviors:
   - fold clothing, stir soup, polish furniture, sweep, rake, and water plants
   - keep a rhythm to music by clapping or playing a rhythm instrument
   - roll yarn

4. To preserve emotions:
   - go on outings to museums
   - engage in musical activities
   - celebrate holidays
5. To practice the client's social skills:
   - take the client out for coffee or for lunch
   - visit with grandchildren
6. To retain the client's habitual behaviors:
   - brush hair, polish nails, and brush teeth
7. To exercise the client's sensory functions:
   - taste various foods
   - look at travel books and at art

Helpful Hints: If the client becomes agitated when playing a game, stop the game and go on to another activity.

REVIEW QUESTIONS

1. Five main areas of concern when caring for the client with AD are:
   a.
   b.
   c.
   d.
   e.
2. List six possible triggers of severe reactions of clients with AD:
   a.
   b.
   c.
   d.
   e.
   f.
3. List four possible causes of incontinence in a client with AD:
   a.
   b
   c
   d.
4. Which of the following are health problems associated with urinary incontinence?
   a. skin breakdown
   b. poor personal hygiene
   c. lack of exercise
   d. poor attention
   e. all of the above

5. Good skin care includes all but which of the following?
   a. dry linen
   b. good nutrition
   c. increased circulation
   d. adequate fluids
   e. use of a bedpan
6. Which of the following members of the health care team should provide input concerning constipation?
   a. nurse
   b. physician
   c. HCA
   d. client with AD
   e. all of the above
7. True or False? Every person has a different time range for normal bowel movements.
8. True or False? Sundowning occurs in every client with AD.
9. True or False? Toys in the bathtub may offer distractions and lower the client's anxiety level.
10. True or False? Clients with AD tend to become malnourished because of their disorientation, inability to handle food, and increased restlessness which raises the body's caloric needs.
11. Unscramble the following key term from the chapter: intcasosdrti _____

CHAPTER 6

Procedures

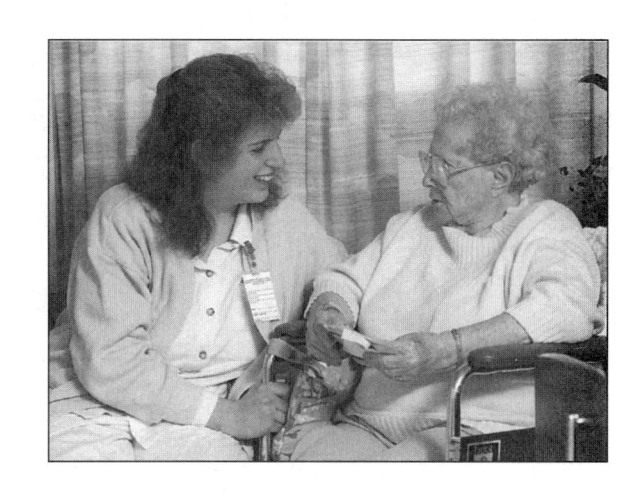

OBJECTIVES Upon reading this chapter and completing the review questions, the home care aide should be able to:
1. Be familiar with skin care and pressure sores.
2. Be familiar with bowel and bladder training.
3. Describe reality orientation and validation therapy.
4. Be familiar with catheter care.

KEY TERMS friction (shearing) reality
perineum validation therapy
pressure sore

INTRODUCTION The HCA who specializes in the care of the client with AD should know the certain procedures that are important to this care. These include skin care, bowel and bladder training, reality orientation, validation therapy, and catheter care.

pressure sore skin breakdown causing redness to tissue destruction

friction (shearing) tearing of skin from rubbing of other tissue or materials

SKIN CARE

Skin care is given to clients with AD to prevent breakdown of the skin which causes **pressure sores**. When there is pressure, or **friction (shearing)** on the skin, breakdown occurs. Because clients with AD have impaired mobility, their risk is higher for pressure sores. Other contributing factors include lack of cleanliness, moisture (perspiration or urine), incontinence, poor nutrition, and soap residue. The skin breaks down in four stages:

Stage I—Redness lasting longer than 30 minutes after pressure is removed. The area may be warm to the touch (see Figure 6-1).

Stage II—The skin is reddened and has a blister or broken area on the surface (see Figure 6-2).

Stage III—Layers of the skin have been destroyed and may or may not include infection (see Figure 6-3).

Stage IV:—Skin is gone and the ulcer is deep into muscle and bone (see Figure 6-4).

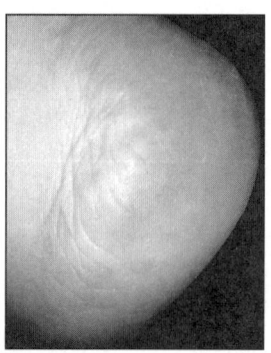

Figure 6-1 First indication of tissue ischemia (Stage I) is redness and heat over a pressure point such as the heel. (Courtesy of Emory University Hospital, Atlanta, GA)

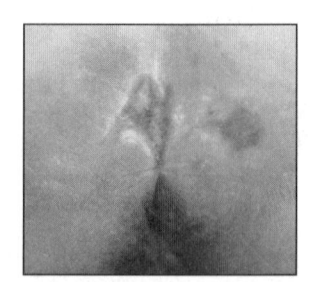

Figure 6-2 In Stage II, the skin is broken and blistered. (Courtesy of Emory University Hospital, Atlanta, GA)

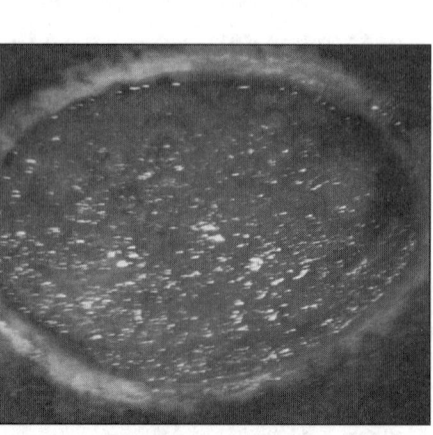

Figure 6-3 In Stage III, all layers of skin have been destroyed. A deep crater has been formed. NOTE: Photo shows right hip. (Courtesy of Emory University Hospital, Atlanta, GA)

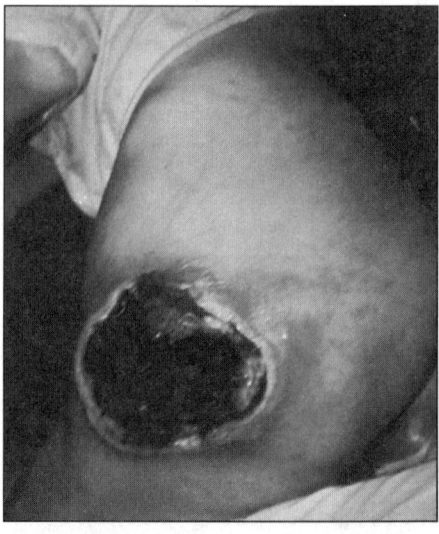

Figure 6-4 In Stage IV, tissue destruction can involve muscle, bone, and other vital structures. (Courtesy of Emory University Hospital, Atlanta, GA)

Seven ways to prevent skin breakdown are:
1. Remove pressure from bony areas.
2. Massage the skin surrounding the area.
3. Keep skin clean and dry.
4. Reposition the client frequently.
5. Remove urine and feces from the skin promptly.
6. Pat skin dry instead of rubbing.
7. Give back massages.

The client's skin should be observed regularly and accurately, especially near pressure points. Figure 6–5 shows the most common sites for pressure sores. The HCA should report any changes in the skin—redness, heat, tenderness, or blisters—immediately. Incontinent clients should be checked for dryness every one to two hours. Depends® and other disposable protective products should be changed frequently. Preventative devices can be used to prevent skin breakdown. Examples include specialty beds, specialty mattresses, sheepskin heel and elbow protectors, and bed cradles. Figures 6–6A, B, C, and D show various preventative devices used to lower the chances of skin breakdown.

HCAs should follow the guidelines set down by their agencies or facilities for special skin care programs. Cleanliness is the main objective, along with careful observation. The HCA and/or the family can apply special creams and ointments as directed by the nurse or the supervisor, and stimulate circulation in the back, buttocks, and bony areas with gentle massage. Refer to Procedure 1 for Special Skin Care and Pressure Sores.

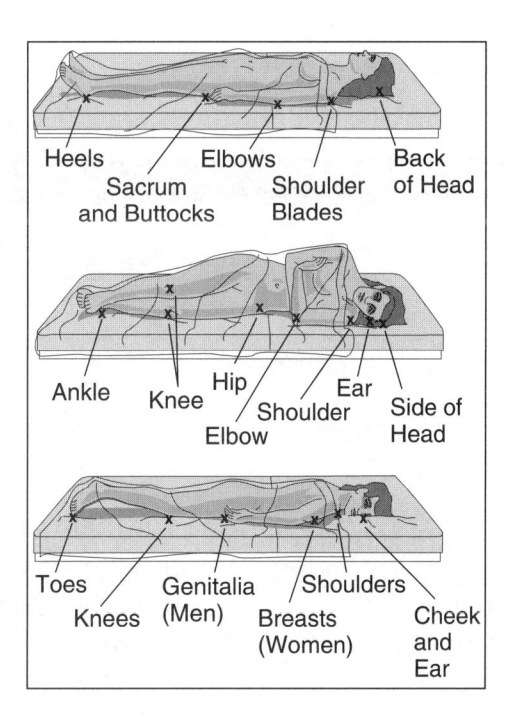

Figure 6–5 Common sites of pressure sores.

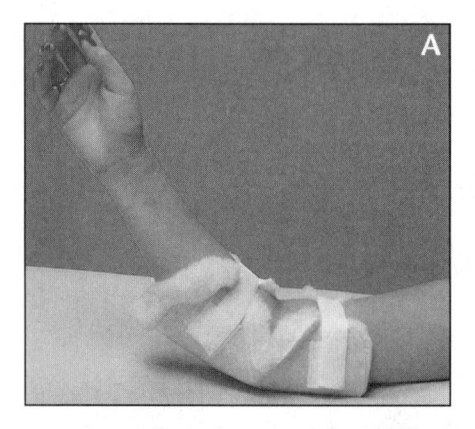

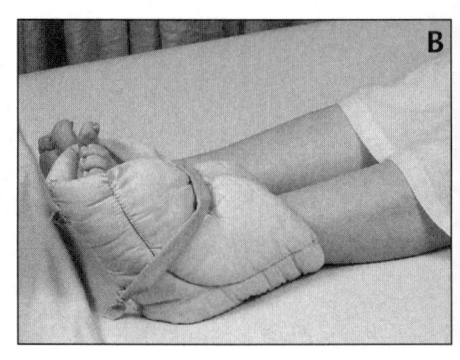

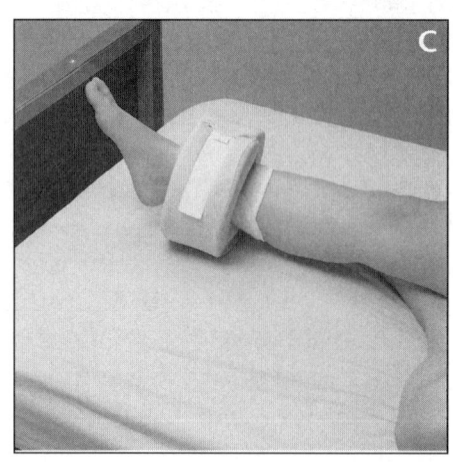

Figure 6–6 A. Pads reduce skin irritation and help prevent pressure sores. (Courtesy of J.T. Posey Co., Arcadia, CA.) B. A heel protector C. Elbow protector

CLIENT CARE PROCEDURE

1 Special Skin Care and Pressure Sores

PURPOSE

- To prevent skin breakdown resulting from pressure and skin irritations
- To use preventive devices
- To prevent friction resulting when skin is in contact with skin or linen

NOTE: Certain clients are at risk for the development of pressure areas leading to sores. Clients at risk are bedridden, obese, very thin, diabetic, paralyzed, and malnourished. A home health aide's role is mainly in the prevention of pressure sore development. Once a pressure sore has developed, the nurse will need to come to the client's home to treat the open area.

CLIENT CARE PROCEDURE, *continued*

1   Special Skin Care and Pressure Sores

ASSISTIVE DEVICES TO PREVENT PRESSURE SORES

1. Air mattress—This is a mattress filled with air. This works by continuously changing the pressure areas on the client's back. One can improvise an air mattress designed for camping instead of buying a medical air mattress.
2. Egg crate mattress—This is a mattress made of foam rubber that is molded like an egg crate. They are inexpensive, but effective in reducing pressure on the skin. You can also purchase one the size of a seat for the client to sit on during the day when up in a chair.
3. Water mattress—This is similar to a regular water mattress used in homes. This mattress is effective in reducing pressure on the skin, but causes problems when transferring clients in and out of bed.
4. Gel foam cushion—This is a special cushion filled with a special solution or gel. This style of cushion is effective in the prevention of pressure sores for a client who sits in a wheelchair for long periods of time.
5. Sheepskin or lamb's wool pads or elbow or heel pads—Lamb's wool pads prevent pressure sores by acting as a barrier between the client's skin and the sheets.
6. Bed cradle—This is a device to keep linens off the client's legs and feet. In the home a client may substitute a box or other device to keep linens off the legs and feet.

SPECIAL CARE TO PREVENT PRESSURE SORES

1. Change client's position at least every 2 hours to reduce pressure on any one area.
2. As quickly as possible, remove feces, urine, or moisture of any kind that might be irritating the skin.
3. Encourage clients who sit in chairs or wheelchairs to raise themselves or change position every 15 minutes to relieve pressure.
4. Encourage client to eat a high protein diet if allowed and drink adequate fluids.
5. Keep the bed linens clean, dry, and wrinkle-free.
6. When bathing clients, use soap sparingly because soap drys skin. Keep skin well lubricated.
7. Watch for skin irritation when applying braces and splints.
8. At the first sign of a reddened area, gently massage area around the reddened area. Report your observations to the nurse superviser.

In addition, the bedbound client should be repositioned every two hours to prevent skin breakdown. The more active client should be encouraged to ambulate as much as is safely possible.

BOWEL AND BLADDER TRAINING

Bowel and bladder training is an important process for clients with elimination dysfunction and incontinence. Some clients have lost all or part of their control and, in some cases, the physician and the nurse might determine that bowel or bladder training would be useful in regaining some or all of this control. Sometimes incontinence can be prevented by offering the bedpan or urinal to the client on a regular basis.

To retrain the bowel the physician might order suppositories to stimulate the rectum to produce a bowel movement. The HCA could be asked to assist the client in inserting the suppository. The HCA should observe the client's ability to control his or her bowels in terms of how long a bowel movement can be retained. Occasionally, enemas will be ordered as part of bowel training. Procedure 2 explains how to give the client an enema but the HCA should first check with the supervisor to determine the agency's policy and procedure for giving enemas. Commercially prepared enemas are usually approved for HCA use. When giving an oil-retention enema the client should retain the oil while in bed, in a quiet position, and hold it for as long as possible.

CLIENT CARE PROCEDURE

2 Giving a Commercial Enema

PURPOSE

- To relieve the client of constipation
- To prepare client for diagnostic tests
- To make the client more comfortable

NOTE: An enema is the technique of introducing fluid into the rectum to remove feces and flatus (gas) from the rectum and colon.

Because enemas distend or dilate the rectum, the client may experience a feeling of urgency in the bowel, that is, a very strong need to empty the bowel as soon as possible.

Enemas can only be given on a doctor's order.

The two commercially prepared enemas are the chemical (often referred to as Fleets) and oil retention enemas. Oil retention enemas are given to soften hard feces in the rectum and are usually followed by a soap solution enema.

CLIENT CARE PROCEDURE, *continued*

2   Giving a Commercial Enema

PROCEDURE

1. Assemble supplies, Figure 6–7.
   gloves
   commercial prepackaged enema
   protective pad
   bedpan (if client is bedridden)
   toilet paper
   lubrication jelly

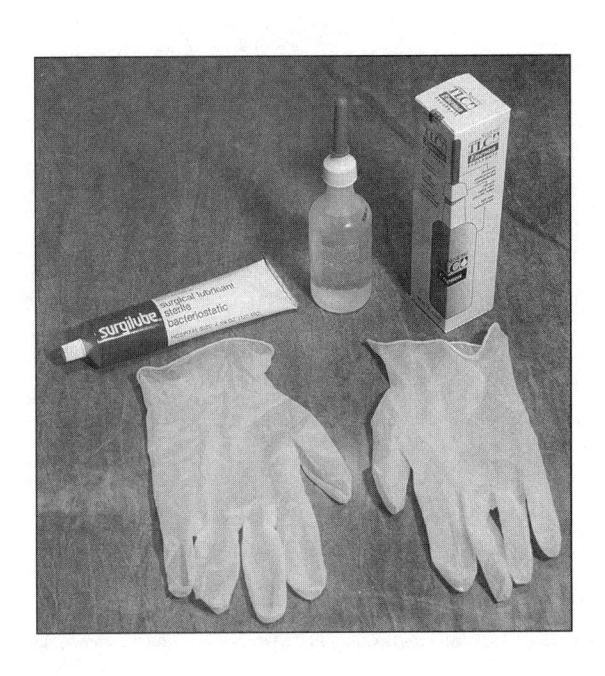

Figure 6–7 Equipment needed to give a commercial enema.

2. Wash hands and put on gloves.
3. Tell client what you plan to do.
4. Provide for the client's comfort and privacy.
5. Have client turn to left side. Turn covers back to expose only the buttocks.
6. Remove cover on tip of enema. Apply extra lubricant to tip to ensure easy insertion.
7. Place protective pad underneath the client's buttocks.
8. Separate the buttocks and insert tip into rectum for at least 3 inches. Tell client to take a deep breath and hold the solution as long as possible. Slowly squeeze the flexible plastic tube, Figure 6–8. This forces the solution to flow evenly into the rectum.

CLIENT CARE PROCEDURE. *continued*

2 Giving a Commercial Enema

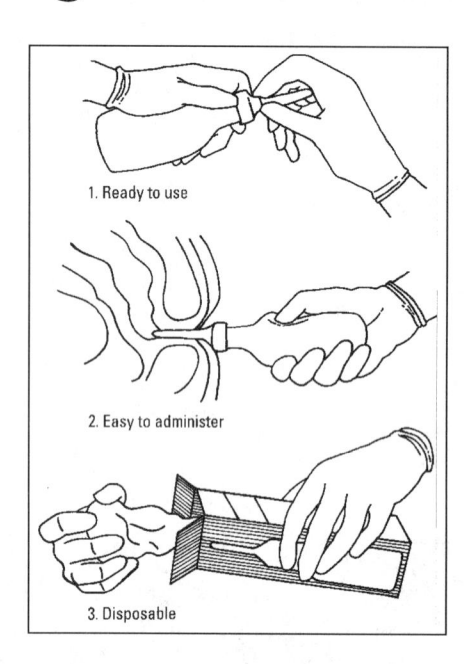

Figure 6–8 Administering a commercial enema. (Courtesy of C.B. Fleet Co., Inc.)

9. Remove enema tip while holding the client's buttocks together.
10. Position client on bedpan, commode, or toilet.
11. After client has expelled feces and enema solution, assist the client in cleaning area around anus and buttocks.
12. Return client to comfortable position. It may be necessary to leave the protective pad in place until the effects of the enema are complete.
13. Remove gloves and wash hands.
14. Record results of enema—color, amount, consistency—10:00 am, Fleet® enema given, good results— large, brown, formed stool.

Some of the areas on which to focus during bowel training include:

1. Observing the bowel pattern by keeping a record of the time and character of each bowel movement.
2. Having the nurse check for fecal impaction.
3. Observing for signs of constipation or diarrhea.
4. Reporting any abdominal or rectal discomfort.

5. Establishing regularity by offering the bedpan or bedside commode at regular times.
6. Administering bowel aides such as suppository or laxatives as prescribed by the physician.
7. Offering a comfortable and private environment for the client to move their bowels.
9. Offering a warm drink to stimulate the bowel movement if the client is unsuccessful.

Adequate fluid intake is an important part of bowel training and in preventing constipation. The HCA and the family should record intake and output on a daily basis. Figure 6–9 shows an example of an intake and output sheet. Sometimes a diet with increased fiber will be ordered by the physician. Bowel training can take up to eight weeks for the client and consistent support from the HCA and the family is crucial. Procedure 3 provides some important tips for bowel training.

Figure 6–9 Sample intake and output sheet.

Date	Time	Method of Adm.	Solution	Intake Amounts Rec'd	Output Urine Amount	Others Kind	Amount
7/16	0700	PO	water	120 mL	500 mL		
	0830	PO	coffee	240 mL			
			or. ju.	120 mL			
	1030	PO	cran. ju.	120 mL			
	1100				300 mL		
	1230	PO	tea	240 mL			
	1400	PO	water	150 mL			
Shift totals	1500			990 mL	800 mL		
	1530	PO	gelatin	120 mL			
	1700	PO	tea	120 mL			
			soup	180 mL			
	2000				512 mL		
	2045					vomitus	500 mL
	2205					vomitus	90 mL
Shift totals	2300			420 mL	512 mL		590 mL
	2345					vomitus	80 mL
	0130	IV	D/W	500 mL			
	0315				400 mL		
Shift totals	0700			500 mL	400 mL		80 mL
24 Hour Totals				1910 mL	1712 mL		670 mL vomitus

CLIENT CARE PROCEDURE

3   Training and Retraining Bowels

PURPOSE

- To train a client to be continent of bowel movement
- To regulate a client to have regular bowel movement

NOTE: Constipation can result from illness, poor eating habits, drug therapy, and lack of exercise. Constipation causes the client added discomfort when it occurs in addition to other physical problems. An individualized bowel program is designed by the health care team for each client. For instance, one client can regulate the bowels by adding prune juice to the diet twice a day. Another client may need to drink daily prune juice but also needs a daily laxative and stool softener by mouth.

Older clients can become overly "bowel conscious" and have a misconception of what normal elimination should be. The frequency of bowel movements may range from three times a day for one person to only once every 2 or 3 days for another. Therefore, the term constipation should not be used to describe a missed movement or two, but only the unusual retention of fecal matter along with infrequent or difficult passage of stony, hard stool.

Among the elderly, constipation is very often encountered. If a client is unable to exercise and move about regularly, bowel action becomes sluggish. Sometimes medications, especially painkillers, can cause constipation. If a client has hemorrhoids, there may be a fear of pain and so the client avoids trying to have a bowel movement. If a client does not have a bowel movement for a few days, the client may develop an impaction. An impaction is a large amount of hard stool in the lower colon or rectum. This is a very painful condition. If a client does develop an impaction, the nurse will need to remove it manually.

PROCEDURE

1. Health care team assesses prior habits of client. If client always had a bowel movement each morning, this would be important to know in planning the client's retraining program.
2. A plan is designed and implemented. Important elements of the plan are:
   - high intake of fiber foods
   - adequate intake of liquids
   - regular exercise
   - toileting client at regular intervals
   - praise by aide of slightest progress of client
   - less reliance on laxatives and enemas
   - privacy for client for bowel movements
3. Follow bowel retraining program developed by the health care team. If plan does appear to be working, note success of program. If plan does not work, report. It is also important to give some suggestions to the health care team of possible solutions for retraining of the client.

Bladder training is most often ordered for clients who have problems with retention of urine. Retraining the bladder takes from six to eight weeks and emotional support from the HCA, and family plays a key role. Figure 6–10 shows an example of a bladder retraining assessment. All members of the team, including the client and the family, have to know the steps in the training program and the role they are to play. The same is true for bowel training as well as bladder training. The client's participation and cooperation is vital to the success of the program.

BLADDER RETRAINING ASSESSMENT
(Reference tags: F315, F316)

CURRENT RESIDENT STATUS

DIAGNOSIS _____ RESIDENT'S AGE _____

RECENT SURGERY? ☐ Yes ☐ No   If Yes, date ___/___/___ and type _____

CURRENT MEDICATIONS (i.e., Diuretics, Psychotropics, etc.) _____

Mental Status and Ability to Communicate	Mobility Status	Vision Status	Right	Left
☐ Alert	☐ Independent	Adequate	☐	☐
☐ Aphasic	☐ Transfer/standing ability	Adequate w/aid	☐	☐
☐ Oriented x____	☐ Wheelchair bound	Poor	☐	☐
☐ Disoriented	☐ Bed rest	Blind	☐	☐
☐ Depressed	☐ Contractures	**Hearing Status**	**Right**	**Left**
☐ Cooperative	☐ Other _____	Adequate	☐	☐
☐ Uncooperative		Adequate w/aid	☐	☐
☐ Slow comprehension		Poor	☐	☐
☐ Other _____		Deaf	☐	☐

BLADDER ASSESSMENT

1. **LENGTH OF INCONTINENCE:** _____ Days _____ Months _____ Years

2. **REASON FOR INCONTINENCE (if known):** _____
   CATHETER: ☐ Yes ☐ No   If Yes, specify type and size _____
   Date inserted ___/___/___ Reason for catheter _____

3. **USUAL VOIDING PATTERN:** Frequency _____ Amt./voiding _____ cc: /24 hrs. _____ cc
   Pattern: ☐ Upon arising ☐ After meals ☐ No apparent pattern ☐ Night time only
   ☐ Other (specify) _____

4. **SYMPTOMS:** (Check all that apply)
   ☐ Voids often in small amounts   ☐ Difficulty stopping stream   ☐ Urgency
   ☐ Fills bladder/voids large amount ☐ Dribbles constantly   ☐ Burning/Pain
   ☐ Unable to void   ☐ Dribbles after voiding   ☐ Edema
   ☐ Difficulty starting stream   ☐ Dribbles while coughing   ☐ Other (specify) _____

5. **HISTORY OF:** ☐ Urinary Disorders ☐ Bladder Disorders ☐ Kidney Disease ☐ Prostate Problems
   ☐ Neurological Disorders ☐ Fecal Impactions ☐ Other (specify) _____

6. **RELIEF AFTER VOIDING:** ☐ Complete ☐ Continued desire to void

7. **BLADDER DISTENDED:** ☐ Yes ☐ No   **EMPTIED BY EXTERNAL STIMULI:** ☐ Yes ☐ No
   If Yes, Check: ☐ Kegel Exercises ☐ Warm water over perineum
   ☐ Other (specify) _____

8. **RESIDUAL URINE:** ☐ Yes ☐ No   If Yes, Amount: _____ cc

9. **PERCEPTION OF NEED TO VOID:** ☐ Present ☐ Diminished ☐ Absent

10. **WELL HYDRATED:** ☐ Yes ☐ No   AVERAGE FLUID INTAKE (24 HRS) _____ cc
    AVERAGE FLUID OUTPUT (24 HRS) _____ cc

    Fluids Preferred _____

NAME—Last	First	Middle	Attending Physician	Chart No.

CFS 6-10HH © 1992 Briggs Corporation, Des Moines, IA 50306 (800) 247-2343
Printed in U.S.A.

BLADDER RETRAINING ASSESSMENT
☐ Continued on Reverse

Figure 6–10 Bladder retraining assessment sheet *(continues)*

EVALUATION FOR BLADDER RETRAINING POTENTIAL

☐ ABLE TO PARTICIPATE IN RETRAINING   EVALUATION PERIOD: _____ TO _____
PLAN: _____

PROVIDE FLUIDS:	FLUIDS SHOULD BE SPACED AS FOLLOWS:				
____ cc every 24 Hrs	☐ 7AM	☐ 11	☐ 3PM	☐ 7	☐ 11PM	☐ 3
____ cc 7-3 shift	☐ 8	☐ 12N	☐ 4	☐ 8	☐ 12MN	☐ 4
____ cc 3-11 shift	☐ 9	☐ 1PM	☐ 5	☐ 9	☐ 1AM	☐ 5
____ cc 11-7 shift	☐ 10	☐ 2	☐ 6	☐ 10	☐ 2	☐ 6

OFFER NO FLUIDS AFTER ____ PM   TOILET FOR VOIDING EVERY ____ Hrs (Day and Evening) ____ Hrs (Night)
(Except as needed for medications)
RECORD RESULTS ON BLADDER RETRAINING RECORD.

☐ UNABLE TO PARTICIPATE IN RETRAINING
REASON: _____

REEVALUATION DATE: _____

COMPLETED BY: _____   ___/___/___
                    Signature/Title   Date

BLADDER RETRAINING PROGRESS NOTES OR REEVALUATION NOTES

DATE	TIME	NOTES - ALL ENTRIES MUST BE SIGNED WITH NAME AND TITLE

NAME—Last   First   Middle   Attending Physician   Chart No.

BLADDER RETRAINING NOTES

Figure 6–10 (continued)

Some of the areas to focus on in bladder retraining are:
1. Fluids should be encouraged in the daytime hours and restricted at night.
2. When offering the bedpan or commode, the client's position is important. The height of the seat and handrails can offer

comfort to the client. Men find it easier to urinate in a standing position.

perineum

3. Additional stimuli may encourage voiding (urinating) such as offering a glass of water, pouring water over the **perineum**, running water in the sink, bearing down to empty the bladder, and placing the client's hand in water.
4. The incontinent client's skin should be cleaned on a regular basis.
5. Offer to assist the client to urinate on a regular schedule (maybe every three to four hours).
6. Keep a careful report of the time and amount of urination on the record and on the Intake and Output sheets.

Procedure 4 fprovides important guidelines for the HCA involved in bladder training a client.

CLIENT CARE PROCEDURE

4 Retraining the Bladder

PURPOSE

- To regain bladder control

PROCEDURE

A home health aide will need to keep a record of how often and how much the client voids throughout the day and night for a few days. Once the client's voiding pattern is known, the nurse supervisor can analyze the client's voiding record and formulate a schedule for the aide to follow. The schedule developed by the nurse will include regularly scheduled times for the aide to have the client drink a measured amount of fluid. After the client has drunk the liquid, the aide notes the time and then 30 minutes later the aide will toilet the client. The aide will need to encourage the client to void each time the client is positioned on the commode or toilet. It is helpful at times to run water from the faucet to give the client an urge to void. Other methods of encouraaging the client to void are to have the client apply light pressure to the bladder area to stimulate the urge to empty the bladder; or have the client lean forward on the toilet to stimulate emptying the bladder. Remember that the client needs to be toileted at regular intervals to prevent accidents. The client will need consistent positive reinforcement to remain dry. At first it may be necessary to take the client to the bathroom every 2 hours; intervals may be lengthened as control is gained. A common cause of incontinence is delay in getting the client to the bathroom. It is of utmost importance to take the client to the bathroom on a regular time schedule. The plan will also call for the aide to maintain the client's fluid intake at about 2500cc/day. The aide should encourage the client to wear regular underwear to enhance the client's self-esteem and to help the client from reverting back to the previous incontinence habit.

Bowel and bladder training are especially difficult with the client who has Alzheimer's disease because the client does not understand what is going on and may not be cooperative. Logging of urination and bowel habits and patterns are very helpful. The HCA will have to rely on the family and caregivers to assist in compiling such a diary.

CATHETER CARE

The risk of infection is very high in clients with catheters in place. To prevent infection, the following measures are important:

1. Make sure the urine is flowing freely through the catheter and that there are no kinks in the tubing.
2. Keep the bag below the level of the bladder to prevent backflow. Attach the bag to the bedframe when the client is in bed.
3. Attach the tubing to the bottom sheet to allow free flow.
4. Secure the catheter to the client's thigh to reduce friction in the urethra.
5. Catheter care (perineal care) should be done every day.
6. The collection bag should be emptied as directed and the urine measured.
7. Report any complaints of pain, burning, or irritation to the supervisor. Chart the color and odor of the urine.
8. Report to the nurse or supervisor if urine is leaking around the catheter.
9. Keep the catheter clean from feces and vaginal drainage.
10. Use a catheter plug or an alcohol protection if the catheter is separated from the drainage tubing.
11. The bag should always be with the client unless a leg bag is applied.
12. Follow good medical asepsis at all times.
13. Always wash hands before and after handling urinary equipment.
14. Always wear personal protective equipment.

Refer to Procedure 5 for guidelines of catheter care but as with all procedures given in this chapter, the HCA should check with the policies and procedures of his or her agency or facility for guidance.

CLIENT CARE PROCEDURE

5 Caring for a Urinary Catheter

PURPOSE

- To clean the area around where the catheter enters the body
- To prevent infection of the urinary tract
- To decrease odors and make the client comfortable
- To maintain closed drainage system correctly

NOTE: A urinary catheter is a tube inserted into the bladder to drain urine. Germs can easily enter the bladder while the catheter is in place. Therefore, cleaning around the urinary opening is important. The catheter is inserted by the nurse. The catheter is replaced weekly or once a month.

The collection bag, tubing, and catheter are referred to as the closed drainage system, Figure 6–11. The system should never be disconnected. The reason the system should not be opened is to prevent germs from entering the system, Figure 6–12. You should never raise the collection bag higher than the client's bladder. Always check to see if the tubing is lying in correct position and not kinked. Always cover bag with a cloth to prevent embarrassment of your client.

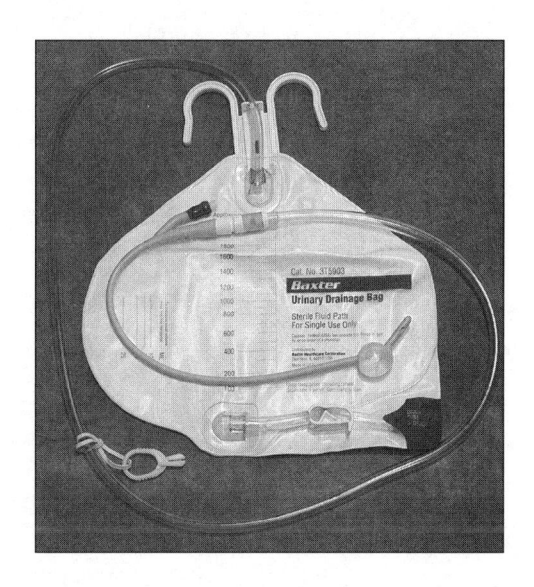

Figure 6–11 Closed drainage system. Note tubing, urine collection bag, and indwelling catheter with bulb inflated.

PROCEDURE

1. Assemble supplies
   gloves
   antiseptic wipes
   basin of warm water
   plastic bag for waste
   cotton-tipped applicators
2. Wash your hands and apply gloves.
3. Tell client what you plan to do.

CLIENT CARE PROCEDURE, continued

5   Caring for a Urinary Catheter

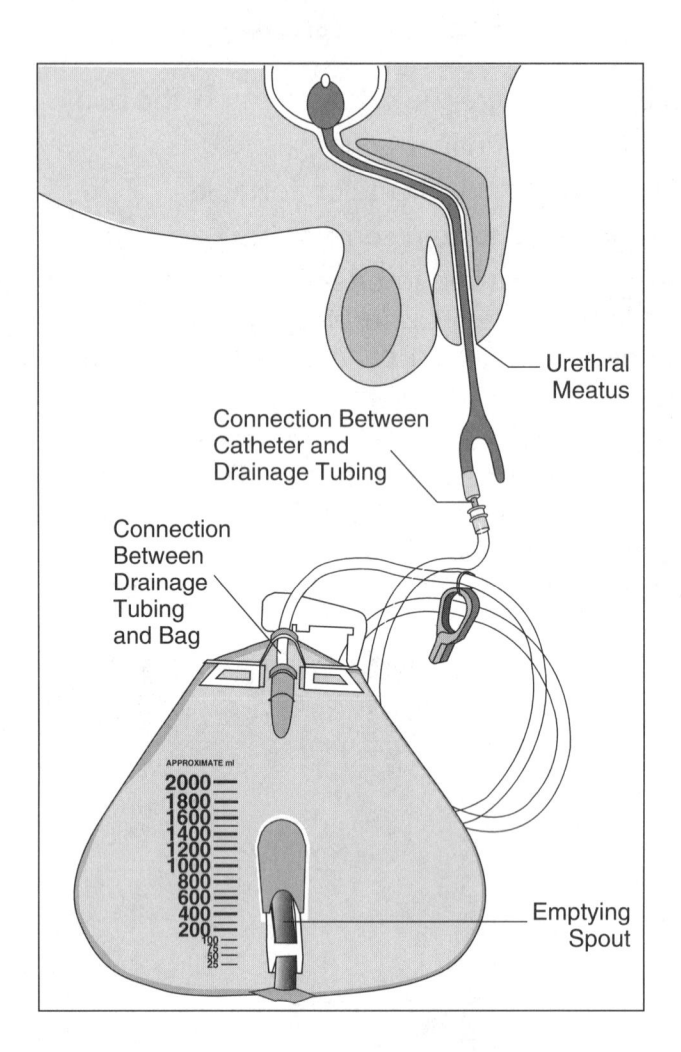

Figure 6–12 Special care must be taken to protect the possible sites of contamination in the closed urinary drainage system.

4. Position client on his or her back. Expose only a small area where the catheter enters the body. Using soap and warm water or antiseptic wipes, wash area surrounding the catheter.
5. Using antiseptic wipes or gauze pads dipped in warm water, wipe the catheter tube. Make only one stroke with each swab or pad. Discard each wipe after one stroke. Start at the urinary opening and wipe away from it. Be careful not to dislodge the catheter. Clean the catheter up to the connection of the drainage tubing.
6. Remove gloves and discard into plastic bag.
7. Check to be sure tubing is coiled on bed, Figure 6–13, and hanging straight down into the drainage container. Check level of urine in the collection bag. Tubing should not be below the collection bag, Figure 6–14. Do not raise collection bag above the level of the client's bladder.

CLIENT CARE PROCEDURE, *continued*

5 Caring for a Urinary Catheter

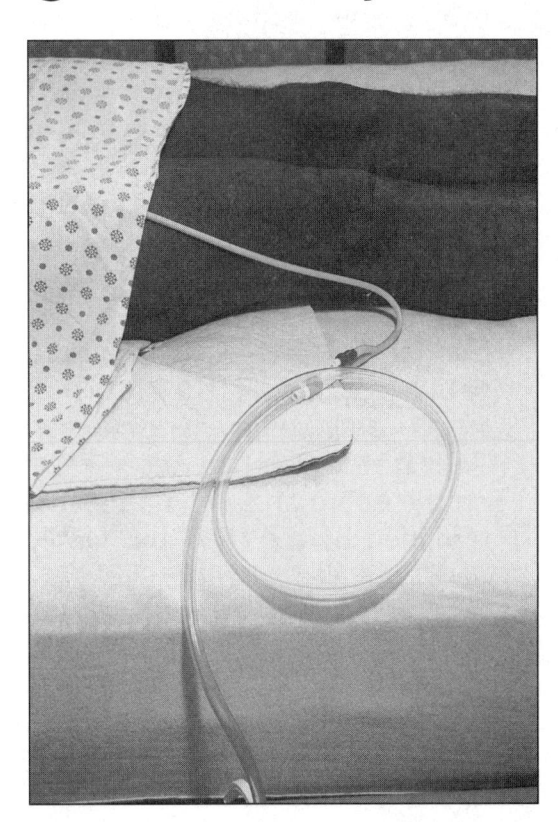

Figure 6–13 Tubing should be placed on top of the leg. The excess tubing should be coiled on the bed.

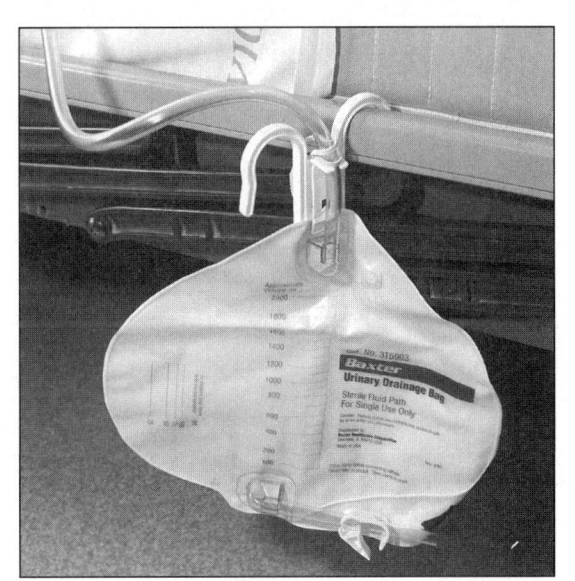

Figure 6–14 The urinary collection bag should be attached to the bed frame. Check to see that the tubing does not fall below the level of the collection bag.

8. Cover client and discard wastes properly.
9. Wash hands.
10. Document procedure and time, your observations, and client's reaction.

reality here and now—not imagined

REALITY ORIENTATION

Reality orientation is useful in the early stages of AD. It is not useful if dementia is severe. Reality orientation helps the mildly or moderately confused person to strengthen his or her contact with the environment and improves the quality of interaction with those around him or her. This is accomplished by helping the client in day-to-day activities using memory aids such as a calendar, a list of daily tasks, written reminders, repeating names frequently, and using other memory stimulation techniques. Forgetting where they are and what task they are doing is very frustrating and dangerous to clients with AD. It is important for them to remain oriented to their surroundings as much as possible. Figure 6–15 is an example of a reality orientation board which contains useful information for the client in the early stages of AD so he or she can maintain a feeling of security.

It is important to know if the client understands the objects on the board and if it is a means of support. This can only be determined by the HCA and family's observations on a day-to-day basis.

A written test often used to test a client's perception difficulty is to ask the client to draw a clock. The more distorted the clock is, the worse the perception problem. The use of reality orientation assists the HCA in determining the mildly confused client's ability to make contact with the environment and provides guidelines for improving the interaction. However, avoid reality testing if it causes anxiety or the client's safety is at risk. Procedure 6 gives steps for the HCA to follow when using reality orientation with a client.

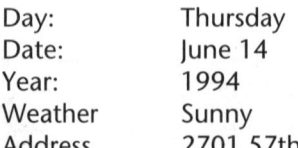

Day:	Thursday
Date:	June 14
Year:	1994
Weather	Sunny
Address	2701 57th Street
City:	Ft. Lauderdale
State:	Florida
Activities:	Bake a cake
	Shampoo hair
Caregiver:	Chris until 10 PM
	Husband, Joe until morning

Figure 6–15 Reality orientation board.

CLIENT CARE PROCEDURE

6   Procedure for Reality Orientation

PURPOSE

- To promote mental awareness to person, place, and time through memory assistance.

PROCEDURE

1. Explain to the family caregivers and other agency personnel what you are going to do, and when
2. Face the patient and maintain eye-to-eye contact if possible
3. Address the patient by name (know what name the patient prefers), speaking slowly and calmly
4. Tell the patient your name and/or show your name tag (it is best to have a picture on the tag)
5. Tell the patient the day, month, year, and time. Then mention where you both are located, and why you are there.
   Example: "Good morning, Mrs. Bass, I'm nurse Gold. It is 9 am on Tuesday, December 27th, 1994. We are in the Sunny Day Home and I will be here for an hour or two to help you with your bath."
6. Touch the patient gently on the hand or shoulder if the supervisor has approved this technique for this particular patient
7. Prepare a reality board and enter the day's information. Discuss the information with the patient and place it in an obvious location.
8. Follow the "guidelines to reality orientation" for communication throughout the period of caregiving.
9. Repeat the reality orientation procedure as frequently as the patient's memory loss requires.
10. When leaving the patient's home it is important to tell the patient your name, that you are leaving, who will be the contact person for the patient and when you will return.

Reality orientation is important because it increases the client's awareness of person, time and place. The following are guidelines for the HCA when conducting reality orientation exercises:

- face the client and speak clearly and slowly
- call the client by name
- state your name and show your name tag frequently
- repeat the date and time frequently during the day
- always explain what you are going to do and why
- give simple answers to the client's questions

Helpful Hints: If reality orientation causes any signs of frustration or anger in the client with AD, it should be avoided. Some clients do not feel comfortable when faced with reality.

Helpful Hints: The specially trained HCA should realize that the client with AD lives in a world that he feels is his or her own "real" world. The HCA should never argue with that concept; instead, the HCA should go along with the client's reality. This causes less frustration for the client.

- ask simple questions and allow enough time for the answer
- keep calendars and clocks visible
- use touch to communicate
- keep familiar items such as pictures around
- maintain the day-to-night cycle by opening curtains during the day and closing them at night
- dress the client in regular clothes during the day rather than allowing him or her to remain in pajamas.
- follow a routine every day for meals, bathing, exercise, television, activities, and recreation
- never rearrange the furniture or the client's belongings

Activity therapy includes comforting activities such as:

- reading to the client.
- watching television with the client (be careful of the program content to avoid anxiety)
- mild exercise like walking
- looking at magazines
- playing simple games

The activities listed above are useful in all stages of AD. Clients seem to prefer simple activities that are offered in one-on-one situations. Children's toys such as blocks or sorting toys are entertaining and activities that appeal to the basic senses of touch, taste, and smell are useful.

Music therapy is also useful. When based on the client's personal tastes in music, it may have a very calming effect.

If the client has hallucinations or inappropriate reactions to normal events, the HCA's response should be to remain calm and reassure the client that the caregiver will protect him or her. What the client sees or hears is believed to be real. If the client becomes violent, the HCA should not put himself or herself in a position of risk.

VALIDATION THERAPY

validation a communication technique used in moderate to severe Alzheimer's clients to increase his or her self-esteem while affirming feelings such as fear and isolation

Validation therapy is a communication technique used for moderate to severe Alzheimer's clients who are disoriented. The goal of the program is to increase the client's self-esteem and, at the same time, validate feelings such as fearfulness and isolation. The basic premise is, if the client wishes to remain in the past, the wish should be honored and no attempt at reorientation should be made. The caregiver accepts the person where he or she is mentally without judgment. This therapy builds trust and security and there is never confrontation or arguments.

Helpful Hints: Validation therapy may replace reality orientation as a more effective therapy in many clients with AD.

Validation therapy can include reminiscence which is remembering and discussing past events and memories, especially pleasant ones. The goal is to emphasize the positive areas in the client's life to build self-esteem.

REVIEW QUESTIONS

1. _____ _____ can prevent pressure sores.
2. _____ _____ is seen in Stage III of skin breakdown.
3. Adequate fluid intake in bowel training can prevent _____.
4. _____ _____ increases the client's awareness of person, time, and place.
5. Which of the following is not included in validation therapy?
    a. wearing pajamas at night only.
    b. honor the client's wish to live in the past.
    c. follow routines for bathing.
    d. keep familiar pictures around.
6. Which are contributing factors to skin breakdown?
    a. poor nutrition
    b. incontinence
    c. poor personal hygiene
    d. all of the above.
7. True or False? Clients with impaired mobility are at higher risk for pressure sores.
8. True or False? Redness over a bony area lasting more than 30 minutes occurs before the stages of skin breakdown begin.
9. True or False? A warm drink may stimulate a bowel movement.

Place a "Y" next to the following items that are memory aides and an "N" next to the ones that are not:

10. _____ calendar
11. _____ orientation board
12. _____ telephones
13. _____ written reminders
14. _____ clocks.
15. Unscramble the following key term from the chapter: lvdataoiin _____

CHAPTER 7

Client and Family Education

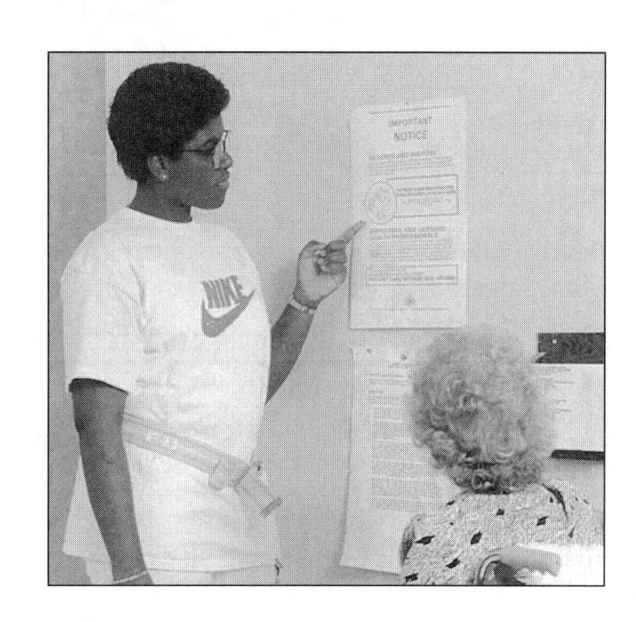

OBJECTIVES Upon reading this chapter and completing the review questions, the home care aide should be able to:
1. Be familiar with specific caregiver education focuses.
2. Describe supportive techniques for families caring for a person with AD.
3. Be familiar with AD community services and support groups.

KEY TERMS coping skills   support groups

INTRODUCTION The nurse on any case is the member of the health care team responsible for client/family education. However, the HCA is often with the client and family more frequently and has more opportunities to offer care, help, and support. This chapter will prepare the HCA to be a knowledgeable caregiver with at least as much information as the client with AD and the family are expected to have. The specially trained HCA will offer assistance and review with the client and family the education offered by the nurse, the dietitian, the medical social worker, and any other professional assigned to the case.

EDUCATING THE FAMILY AND THE CLIENT WITH AD

Because the client with AD is usually not capable of being taught about his or her illness in moderately severe to severe cases, education is usually directed toward the family, particularly the caregiver or caregivers. There are several important areas the nurse should explain when educating the family and the HCA should support these teachings in subsequent visits.

The client with AD and the caregiver should understand the nature of the disease. The signs and symptoms of complications that could occur and the effect of the disease on mobility and memory are basic to the education of the family concerning the disease process. After completing this education training, the HCA should be able to answer some basic questions concerning the disease process.

The nurse will leave written materials with the family. The HCA can obtain more information from the nurse, the supervisor, or support organizations. The family should be able to define Alzheimer's disease and know the signs and symptoms of the three stages of AD.

The HCA's four primary goals of the education and support training are to:

1. Learn caregiving skills to provide care at home.
2. Know where to get the telephone helplines.
3. Become aware of techniques and the importance of stress management for himself or herself.
4. Be familiar with community and professional resources and support.

When the family asks the HCA questions about the disease process of AD, there should be printed materials left by the nurse to which he or she can refer. The HCA should become familiar with these printed materials available from the agency regarding AD.

The caregiver should be taught communication skills by the nurse that are specific to helping that person communicate with the client with AD. The Alzheimer's Association has an excellent pamphlet in their caregivers series entitled "Communicating with the Alzheimer's Client." This is a helpful addition to the family's educational material. The HCA should reinforce the communication skills taught by the nurse. The HCA who takes this specialty training program will know the techniques of communicating

> **Helpful Hints:** The HCA is not expected to educate the family but should be able to answer simple questions the caregiver or family might have concerning the education plan initiated by the nurse.

with the client with AD and serve as a role model for the family. The family will learn from watching the HCA's responses to the client's behavior on a day-to-day basis.

Safety in the home environment is a twenty-four-hour problem and the family should be instructed as to how to maintain a safe and healthy environment for the client. The nurse assesses the home for safety and establishes a program for safety changes. The HCA is expected to help facilitate the changes and observe the results. Figure 7–1 shows the HCA explaining safety procedures to the family. Any safety changes not made by the family that the HCA feels could put the client at risk should be reported to the supervisor.

A well-balanced diet is important and the family will be instructed by the dietitian or the nurse concerning shopping, preparation, and storage of nutritious and fresh foods in order to maintain the optimal level of nutrition for the client. The HCA will be an asset to the home care team by offering suggestions and observing whether or not the family is participating as instructed by the nurse. It is important that the client be weighed on every visit and the weight recorded so that weight loss can be reported to the physician. In some situations, when time permits, the HCA may prepare meals, particularly as a relief to the caregiver. The HCA should be familiar with any special diets that have been ordered for the client. The most common of these diets consists of soft, chewable foods, high-calorie supplements, and high-fiber foods.

Helpful Hints: The HCA should ask the client with AD or the family to suggest some of his or her favorite foods that are nutritious and easy to eat so that they can be included in the client's diet.

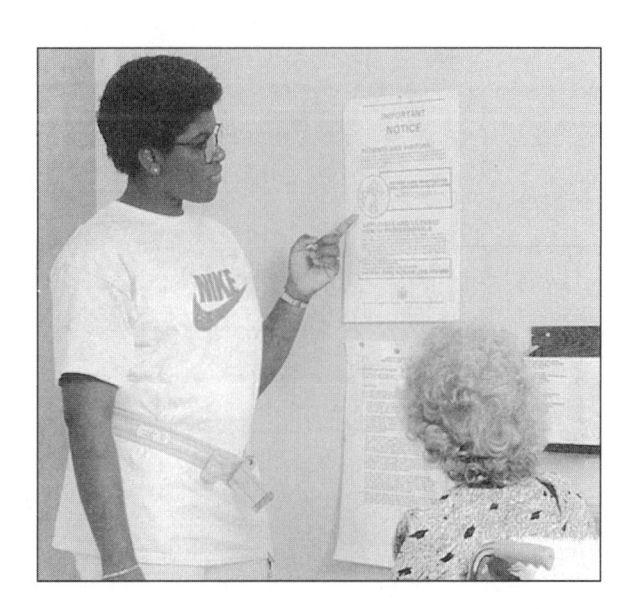

Figure 7–1 The HCA should support the nurse's teaching concerning safety.

The written material provided to the family should include stress relieving techniques as well as relaxation methods for the caregiver. As previously mentioned, controlling the stress level of the caregiver is important in caring for the client with AD.

If bowel or bladder training is implemented, the family needs instructions concerning their role in the program. The nurse will instruct them on how to record information on the log and to use the same techniques implemented in the procedure. The HCA will assist the family to begin and record this training program at home. The success of the program will depend on the family's understanding that it is a twenty-four-hour plan, and without their cooperation, the plan will fail.

It is important for the physician or nurse to instruct the family to accept the client and his or her behavior as deterioration occurs. They must be reassured that feelings of guilt, anger, and resentment are common. The HCA will be the one to listen as the family expresses these feelings. They should be encouraged to take time away from the client by attending a **support group** and to plan for respite, either by hiring in-home day care or placing the client in a temporary overnight facility. The HCA will observe the family for signs of stress and report these signs to the supervisor while encouraging the family to seek relief and support. Figure 7–2 shows the numerous relationships involved when caring for a client with AD.

Other ways the HCA can assist the nurse in the education of the family includes:

1. Follow-up on safety instructions to see that changes that were recommended by the nurse have been made.
2. Assisting the family to plan nutritious meals as ordered by the physician. The HCA should emphasize the importance of the client's diet and assist the family to read food labels and prepare foods that are easy to eat. The HCA should also ensure that the client's dentures fit properly.

support groups persons who have interests or problems in common and offer each other guidance and assistance

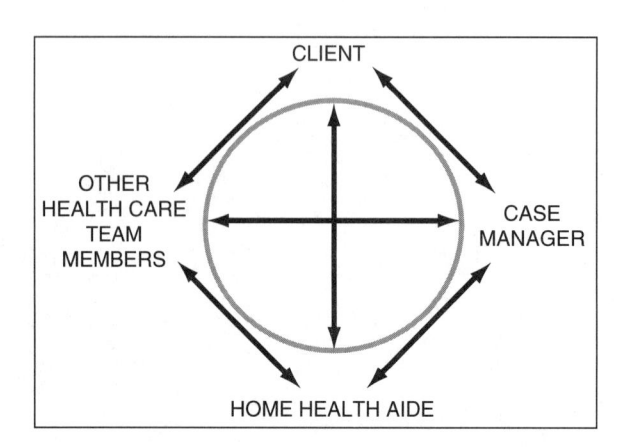

Figure 7–2 Learning to handle relationships is part of the HCA's job.

3. Follow-up on bowel and bladder training programs and support the family in recording and logging bowel movements and voidings.
4. Demonstrating good communication responses as taught by the nurse and this training text. The HCA is a role model for the family and from whom they will learn.
5. Demonstrating appropriate responses to the client's abnormal behaviors. The family should learn that they can control their responses but not the client's behavior.
6. Encouraging and demonstrating reality orientation, the use of distractions, music therapy, and validation therapy as appropriate to each case.
7. Assisting the family members to care for themselves by taking time off and using stress reduction techniques when appropriate.

The education of the family caring for a client with AD is as important as the client's care. Without the family's support and care, the client with AD would most certainly not exist in any state of health or security and deterioration would occur more rapidly and severely. Figure 7–3 shows the caring attitude an HCA must have when caring for the client with AD.

Friends and visitors should be encouraged but at a convenient time for the family and client. Visitors should arrive in small groups and terminate the visit if the client appears anxious or tired. Visitors should be informed that AD clients have set routines and visits should never be scheduled during normal rest pe-

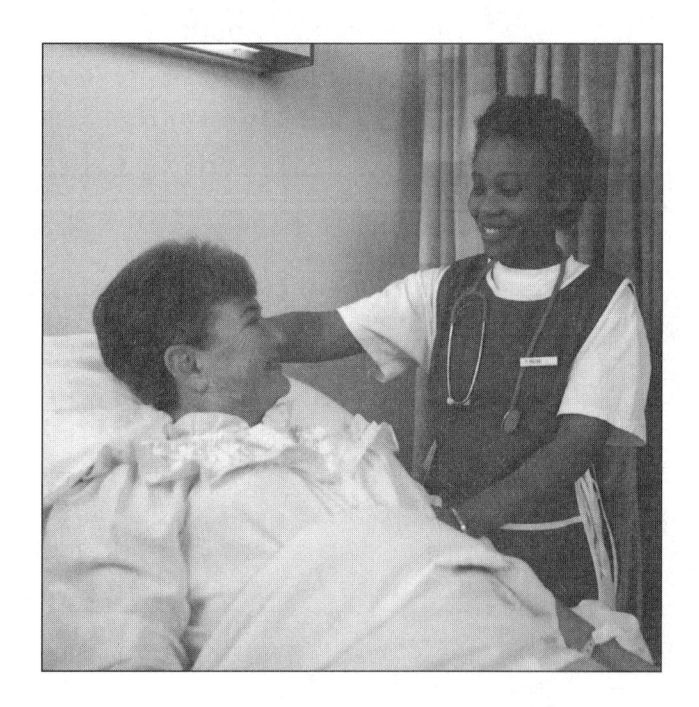

Figure 7–3 The facial expression of the HCA shows a caring attitude.

coping skills ability to use learned skills to handle a situation

riods. Visitors should be encouraged to bring small gifts and familiar pictures or objects from the client's past. Regular visitors should be included in the activities and games the client likes. The HCA should observe the client for responses, good or bad, from all visitations.

The family must be given **coping skills** and the names of community support services available in their area. Community support is any assistance, including informational, emotional, and physical, that a person receives as a result of community and social ties. Friends can also become involved to help the family caring for a client with AD.

THE ALZHEIMER'S ASSOCIATION

Founded in 1980 by family caregivers, the Alzheimer's Association has more than 200 chapters nationwide providing programs and services to assist Alzheimer families in their communities. The Alzheimer's Association is the leading funding source for Alzheimer research after the federal government.

Information on Alzheimer's disease, current research, patient care, and assistance for caregivers is available from the Alzheimer's Association. For more information or the location of the chapter nearest the client, call (800) 272-3900 or write to the Alzheimer's Association, 919 North Michigan Avenue, Suite 1000 Chicago, IL 60611-1676. Their E-mail address is info@alz.org.

Other community services and support programs for Alzheimer's families include:

- Respite Services and Care Centers Helpline
- local support groups
- Wanderer's Identification Programs
- AD Chapter newsletters
- Extended Care and Day Care Families

MATERIALS FOR YOUNG PEOPLE

Alzheimer's disease effects entire families including children and young adults. A variety of materials, created for children of all ages, specifically address the informational needs of young people. Some of the resources that are available are:

Grandpa Doesn't Know It's me by Donna Guthrie, illustrated by Katy Keck Arnsteen, 1986. Twenty-six pages available from the Alzheimer's Association Office Services, 919 North Michigan Avenue, Suite 1000, Chicago, IL 60611 (312) 335-5796 or from the local chapter: order number ED 103Z—$5.95. Lizzie is a young girl whose grandfather has Alzheimer's. She reminisces about enjoyable experiences she has shared with her grandfather and demonstrates how she and her family cope with the changes and emotions they experience. This book is intended for students preschool through fourth grade.

Danger at Rock River: The Neuro Explorers in a Memorable Misadventure by Dane Chetkovich, illustrated by T. Lewis, 1993. Thirty-eight pages available from BrainLink Materials, 1709 Dryden, Suite 545, Houston, TX 77030 (713) 798-8200—$7.50. In a series of exciting adventures, a group of children discover how the brain works. One boy's grandfather has Alzheimer's, and at one point in the story, the gentleman wanders into the woods and becomes lost. The story features positive visits to a nursing home and addresses questions frequently asked by children. This book is intended for elementary schools students.

Someone I Love Has Alzheimer's. One video cassette, 17 minutes and curriculum guide. Available from InJoy Productions, 3970 Broadway, Suite B4, Boulder, CO 80304 (800) 326-2082—$24.95 for home use, $49.95 for professional use. This video, produced by the Alzheimer's Association's Eastern Massachusetts Chapter and narrated by actress Shelley Fabres, features interviews with children who share their thoughts, feelings, and some practical advice about coping with Alzheimer's.

Just for the Summer. One video cassette, 1990, 29 minutes. Available from Churchill Films, 12210 Nebraska Avenue, Los angeles, CA 90025 (800) 334-7830—$129.95. A high school student believes his summer is ruined when he discovers his grandmother, who has Alzheimer's, will move into the family's home. But in time, he comes to understand her illness and finds ways to connect with her. The video is aimed at those twelve years of age and older. A *Just for the Summer* curriculum manual (1991, 52 pages) is available from the Alzheimer's Association Office Services 919 North Michigan Avenue, Suite 1000, Chicago,IL 60611 (312) 335-5796, or from your local chapter—order number ED 251ZCM. $25.00.

Talking with Children and Teens About Alzheimer's Disease: A Question and Answer Guidebook for Parents, Teachers, and Caregivers by J. M. McCrea, 1994, 75 pages. Available from Generations Together, University of Pittsburgh, 121 University Place, Suite 300, Pittsburgh, PA 15260 (412) 648-7150—order number 138. $15.00. This guidebook provides parents and health care professionals with strategies for helping young people understand Alzheimer's disease. Sections include tips for communicating with preschoolers, school-age children, and teenagers. "Talking points" on personality change, behavior, and memory loss are included.

These reviews were prepared by the staff of the Association's Benjamin B. Green-Field Library and Resource Center. A more extensive reading list of materials for children and young adults is available from the library at (312) 335-9602. All revised materials are part of the Green-Field Library collection.

REVIEW QUESTIONS

1. The _____ is the member of the health care team responsible for client-family education.
2. The _____ is the person who often spends the most time with the client and family and reinforces education.
3. The Alzheimer's Association has more than _____ chapters nationwide providing programs and services to assist Alzheimer families in their communities.
4. The HCA's four primary goals of education and support are to:
   a. Learn _____ _____
   b. Know _____ _____
   c. Become aware of _____
   d. Be familiar with _____
5. Which of the following should be included in the educational program of the client with AD and his or her family?
   a. safety in the home.
   b. well-balanced diet.
   c. communication skills
   d. validation therapy
   e. all of the above
6. True or False? The education of the family caring for a client with AD is as important as the client's care.
7. True or False? The family will not play a role in bladder training.
8. True or False? A well-balanced diet is never included as part of the family's education.
9. True or False? The HCA is a role model.
10. True or False? The Alzheimer's Association is only concerned about the person with AD.
11. Unscramble the following key term from the chapter: gnopic lsklis _____ _____

CHAPTER 8

The Caregiver

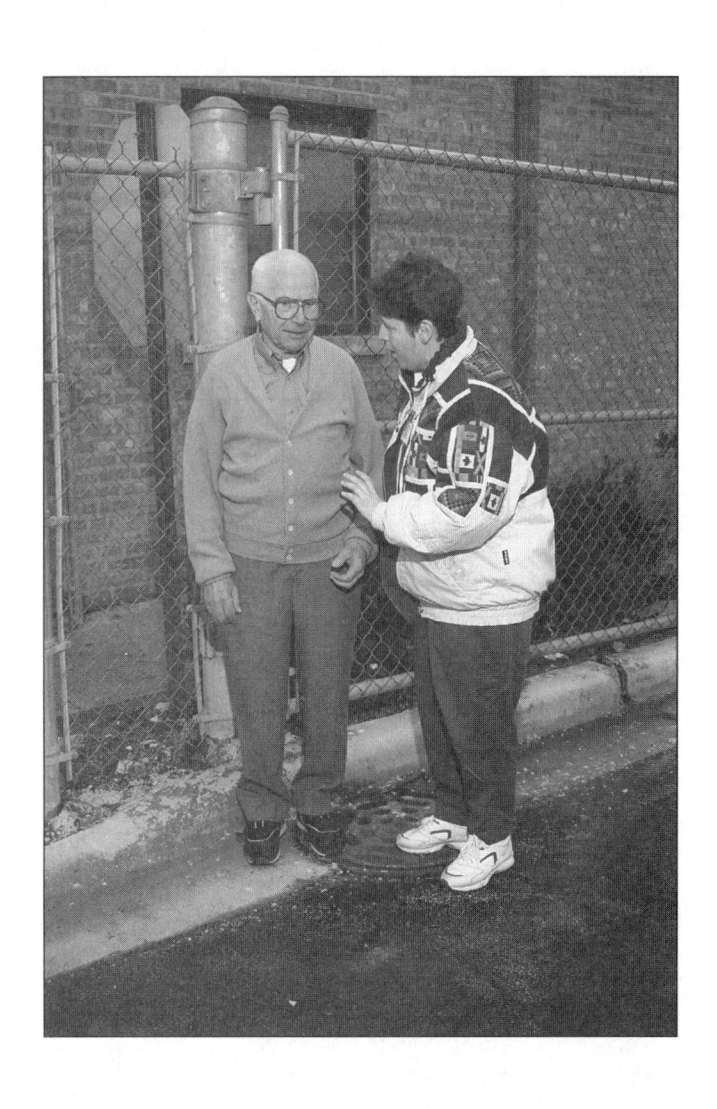

OBJECTIVES

Upon reading this chapter and completing the review questions, the home care aide should be able to:

1. Define the term caregiver and the implications involved in caring for a client with Alzheimer's disease.
2. Recognize the stresses involved in caring for a client with Alzheimer's disease and learn ways to manage them.
3. Be familiar with caring techniques for caregivers of clients with Alzheimer's disease.
4. Recognize human needs based on Maslow's hierarchy of needs as they apply to caregivers, including HCAs.

KEY TERMS

caregiver
health caregiver
primary caregiver
prognosis
respite
self-esteem
stress
stress management
technique

INTRODUCTION

This chapter gives the HCA an insight into the stresses and demands made on the persons or family members who care for a loved one with AD. As the support person and role model for the family, the HCA must have insight, knowledge, and understanding of these important persons. This chapter also looks at the HCA as a caregiver and discusses the unusual stresses that health caregivers experience. Caring suggestions offer possible assistance to all AD caregivers.

CARING FOR THE CLIENT WITH AD

Caring for most clients with AD is a twenty-four-hour-a-day task. In fact, one famous book written by a woman caring for a family member with AD is entitled *The 36 Hour Day* which was exactly how long this caregiver felt a day of caring for a client with AD seemed. The health care team must educate the family as well as themselves to prepare for the strength and skills required to meet this special challenge.

A basic understanding and knowledge of the disease is necessary for persons who are caring for a client with AD. Knowing why behavior is occurring, knowing what to expect, preparing as much as possible for appropriate responses, and using coping techniques are invaluable to the caregiver. A sense of some control over the situation is important because the client does not feel in control and the caregiver must have a sense of security and control from day to day. In many ways, the mental well-being and health of the caregiver is as important as that of the client.

Helpful Hints: The HCA must listen to, and show appreciation and caring for, the family because the client with AD is unable to do so.

THE CAREGIVER

The term **caregiver** usually refers to the person living in the home with the client with AD who is primarily responsible for the care the client is given from day to day. The HCA or other trained health care person who cares for the client is the **health caregiver**. Because these clients progress from needing supervision and limited assistance to requiring total care, the caregiver of the client with AD ultimately will have a twenty-four-hour-a-day, seven-day-a-week responsibility. In addition, the family caregiver

caregiver the person in the home who is responsible for day-to-day client care

health caregiver the trained health care person caring for the client

primary caregiver

often provides much of the care to other members of the family. Sometimes the caregiver is called the **primary caregiver** if the client is at home. The primary caregiver is whoever is responsible for the overall well-being of the client every day, not part-time or by visit. This person is usually a family member or a significant other who lives with the client. Figure 8–1 shows a client with AD and his wife. If the client resides in a facility, there is no primary caregiver unless one person is assigned to care for the client every day.

The role of a primary caregiver is important because a trusting relationship must be established between this person and the client. This trust is built on unwritten promises or an unwritten contract that states to the client with AD:

1. I care about you.
2. I want to assist you.
3. You can depend on me.
4. I will do my best.
5. If I need help I will get it.
6. I will take care of myself and you, too.

Caregivers must be cautioned that the family member with AD shows symptoms of a disease and that his or her behavior should not be taken personally. The words, actions, anger, and uncooperative attitude are really the illness speaking, not the person. The HCA in a situation such as this should devote a percentage of time helping the caregiver as well as the client. Each person's ability to cope with a task as great as caring for a client with AD is different.

Helpful Hints: The HCA should encourage the primary caregiver to be honest about his or her coping abilities.

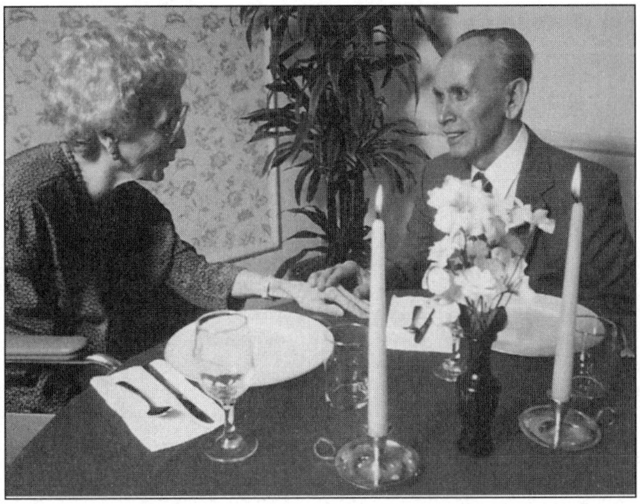

Figure 8–1 The primary caregiver is usually a significant other who lives with the client with AD. (Courtesy of Country Park Health Care Center, Long Beach, CA)

respite periods rest from tasks and roles

All caregivers need **respite** or periods of rest from their tasks and role in order to regain strength and energy. This may be a day off or a month off, whichever is appropriate. However, scheduling coverage for periods of respite is itself a challenge and that is when experienced health caregivers such as HCAs may play a vital part. The family caregiver must feel comfortable that the loved one will be well cared for before a guilt-free respite can be successful. Support groups and resources offer valuable opportunities for family caregivers to express bottled-up emotions and share experiences with other persons in similar situations. The caregiver can find others who truly understand.

When outside help is called in, many times the family is in a crisis. The caregiver may even be ill from the strain. There is sometimes guilt associated with admitting that the task is too great for one caregiver. The HCA must never add to these feelings by being critical or nonsupportive of the caregiver.

Family caregivers who provide care for a family member with AD in the home usually have no training. Adult children are usually the caregivers for disabled parents. Because many women are working, caregivers have become spouses, daughters, sisters, nieces, and even friends. Eighty-five percent of all caregivers are women who also have a multitude of other responsibilities, including a family of their own. In addition, the number of caregivers will increase in the future because the number of persons needing care in the home will increase from six million to seven or eight million by the year 2000. For this reason, the stress of the caregiver is an important consideration. **Stress** is mental, physical, or emotional tension, strain, or distress. Some of the stresses a family caregiver experiences include:

stress emotional, physical or mental strain or tension

- physical strain of caring for the disabled client
- isolation
- loss of personal time
- lack of sleep
- financial expense of caring for a client with AD
- strained family relationships
- emotional impact of watching a loved one decline
- frustration with the inappropriate behavior of the client with AD

The different stresses on caregivers have been studied and the following predictors or indicators have been identified as causes. These include:

- the degree of mental and physical impairment of the client with AD
- the amount of social and emotional support received

- the number of hours per week and number of years spent as caregiver
- the amount of recreation outside the home
- physical and mental health of the caregiver
- previous relationships between the client and family caregiver

The entire family unit is under stress when there is a disabled or dysfunctional elderly member of the family in the home. Alzheimer's disease creates personality changes that are very negative in nature, and all family members eventually respond with anger and resentment.

The HCA is in a good position to observe the caregiver in the home environment. The HCA should observe the stress level of the caregiver and the family and note signs that indicate the caregiver needs relief which include:

- denial about the **prognosis** (probable outcome)
- feelings of exhaustion, anger, and resentment
- a loss of loving and caring emotions toward the client
- destructive behavior such as overeating, undereating, drug abuse, alcohol abuse, and elderly abuse
- withdrawal from friends and social activities
- mental and physical health problems
- anxiety
- refusing outside assistance
- showing unrealistic goals
- family breakdown and poor communication
- feelings of inadequacy and isolation
- depression and poor coping skills
- irritability and sleep problems
- forgetting to do tasks

To grown children struggling to balance the demands of career and family, a sick parent can raise stress to unmanageable levels. When a parent is diagnosed with AD, it is common for a son or daughter to assume the role of caregiver within his or her own home. Although committed to the loved one's care, the point may come when the adult child can no longer bear the physical and emotional demands without risking his or her own psychological well-being and that of the whole family.

The HCA may be called upon to relieve the family by assuming the caregiving role for varying lengths of time, from a two-hour visit to a twelve- or twenty-four-hour day. Four basic rules for anyone caring for a client with AD include:

1. Keep a recent photograph of the client handy for emergency use should he or she wander off.

Helpful Hints: It is important for the HCA to be aware of his or her own stress levels as well as those of the family.

prognosis probable outcome

2. When the client asks "What day is this?" do not respond with a questions such as "What day do you think it it?" Instead, respond by giving the correct day.
3. Remain calm and do not argue with the client.
4. Constantly reassure the client that he or she is safe.

The HCA, along with the other members of the home care team, should encourage the family caregiver to seek as much relief time as possible from other family members, friends, the church, and community resources. The HCA, when called upon to relieve the caregiver in the home, should encourage the whole family to leave the residence during that time frame and seek activities that will relieve stress.

Stress management is an important element in the caregiving role. It means a deliberate attempt to control stress through acceptable techniques of stress reduction. The family, as well as the HCA, need to understand the importance of stress management to control their stress levels while caring for the client with AD. Common physical signs of excessive stress include:

- increased heart rate
- elevated blood pressure
- rapid, shallow respirations
- increased muscle tension
- tight muscles
- increased perspiration

Frequently, physical exercise can be a great stress reliever. The exercise can be as simple as a scheduled walk or as extensive as aerobic workouts. All exercise programs should be monitored by a physician.

Stress management begins with recognizing that there is stress involved in the caregiver role. Once the HCA has recognized and accepted this fact, stress management techniques should be utilized several times a day to promote relaxation. Some of these techniques include:

1. Deep breathing exercises.
2. Ten-to-one count. Inhale by taking a deep breath, then exhale slowly, counting backward from ten to one while saying "I feel more relaxed than I did at the previous number.
3. Active progressive relaxation such as tensing the muscles in the arms, shoulders, back, and legs for ten to fifteen seconds, then completely relaxing them for twenty to thirty seconds.
4. Passive progressive relaxation. Start at the toes and move up the body to the head, telling each body part to relax as you get to it.

---

stress management deliberate attempt to control stress through acceptable techniques of stress reduction

5. Music therapy which includes listening to music that has a relaxing effect (different for each person).
6. Bio-feedback done in a physician's office with a monitoring device.

Tension relievers can be utilized in a very short period of time. The following tension relievers can be done in a minute or less:

- curling and uncurling the toes
- visualizing a vacation
- meditating on somebody or on an object for one minute
- writing down some goals for the day
- thinking of something that makes one feel happy
- complementing a person
- yawning and stretching to get oxygen to the brain
- breathing deeply
- focusing on a body part that is tense, thereby relaxing it
- taking one's own pulse
- massaging the hands
- delegating tasks

The Alzheimer's Association has published the following ten easy ways to help a family caring for a client with AD:

1. Keep in touch. Maintain contact with family members. A card, a call, or visit all mean a great deal. Family members, including the client with Alzheimer's, benefits from visits or calls. Continue to send cards, even if there is no response. It is a simple but important way to show caring.
2. Do little things; they mean a lot. When cooking, make extra portions and drop off a meal. Surprise the caregiver with a special treat such as a rented movie, an audio tape of last week's church service, or a gift certificate for a massage or dinner out.
3. Give the caregiver a break. Everyone needs a little time for himself or herself. Offer to stay with the client so family members can run errands, attend support group meetings, or take a short trip. Even if the caregiver does not leave the house, this provides some personal time. Chances are the person with Alzheimer's will also enjoy the break.
4. Be specific when offering assistance. Most friends are good about saying they are available to "do anything," but many caregivers find it hard to ask for something specific. Have the family prepare a "to do" list of hard-to-get-to projects (for example, laundry, dusting, yard work, medical bills). Figure out what can be done, then dedicate some time—on a

weekly or monthly basis—to helping the family tackle some of these tasks.

5. Be alert. Learn about Alzheimer's and how it impacts the family. Most people with Alzheimer's "wander" at some point and could become lost in their own neighborhoods. Know how to recognize a problem and respond. Take time to learn about other common behaviors and helpful care techniques.
6. Provide a change of scenery. Plan an activity that gets the whole family out of the house. Make a reservation at a restaurant and ask for a table with some privacy. Be sure to include the person with Alzheimer's if the caregiver feels it is appropriate. If not, make arrangements for someone to stay at home.
7. Learn to listen. Sometimes those affected by Alzheimer's simply need to talk to someone. Ask family members how they are doing and encourage them to share. Be available when the caregiver is free to talk without interruptions. Try not to question or judge; support and accept instead.
8. Care for the caregiver. Encourage caregivers to take care of themselves. Pass along useful information and offer to attend a support group meeting with them. Local chapters of the Alzheimer's Association have information available, sponsor telephone "Helplines," and support groups in the area.
9. Remember all family members. The person with Alzheimer's appreciates visits, even if he or she is unable to show it. Spouses, adult children, and even young grandchildren are all affected in different ways by a relative's AD. Be attentive to their needs.
10. Get involved. Unless a prevention or cure is found, fourteen million Americans will have Alzheimer's disease in the coming years. Make a contribution to the Alzheimer's Association or volunteer at your local chapter.

Some caregiver tips for the family caregiver when the HCA is not present to assist them in their tasks and reduce stress include:

1. Read to the client to keep him or her in touch with reality.
2. Look at picture albums to help recall past memories.
3. Tape personal messages to prevent loneliness. Include favorite songs or poems.
4. Assign or assist with simple household tasks such as dusting or sweeping to make him or her feel useful and less dependent.
5. Lay out clothing in the morning to remind the client to dress for the day.

6. Prepare nutritious and easy-to-eat snacks and leave in places that are easy for the client to access.
7. Keep a schedule so that tasks become routine including activities and medications.
8. Assign family members to specific times and tasks so caregivers have respite periods.
9. Encourage self-care to build client **self-esteem**.

self-esteem how a person feels about themselves and their importance and value

WAYS TO REDUCE CAREGIVER STRESS

The Alzheimer's Association has also suggested the following ten ways in which to reduce caregiver stress:

1. Get a diagnosis as soon as possible. Symptoms of AD appear gradually, and if a person seems physically healthy it is easy to ignore unusual behavior or attribute it to something else. See a physician when AD warning signs are present. Some dementia symptoms are treatable. Once the diagnosis is made, the family will be better able to manage the present and plan for the future.
2. Know what resources are available. Become familiar with AD care resources in the community. Adult day care, in-home assistance, visiting nurses, and Meals-on-Wheels are just some of the community services that can help. The local Alzheimer's Association chapter is a good place to start.
3. Become an educated caregiver. As AD progresses, different caregiving skills and abilities are necessary. Care techniques and suggestions available from the Alzheimer's Association can help the caregiver better understand and cope with many of the challenging behaviors and personality changes that often accompany AD.
4. Get help. Trying to do everything alone leaves the caregiver exhausted. The support of family, friends, and community resources can be an enormous help. If assistance is not offered, ask for it. If the caregiver has difficulty asking for assistance, have someone become an advocate for him or her. If stress becomes overwhelming, do not be afraid to seek professional help. Alzheimer's Association support group meetings and Helplines are a good source of comfort and reassurance.
5. Take care of yourself. Caregivers frequently devote themselves totally to those for whom they care, and in the process, neglect their own needs. Watch your diet, exercise, and get plenty of rest. Use respite services to take time off for shopping, a movie, or an uninterrupted visit with a friend.
6. Manage the level of stress. Stress can cause physical problems (blurred vision, stomach irritation, high blood pressure)

and changes in behavior (irritability, lack of concentration, loss of appetite). Note any symptoms. Use relaxation techniques that work and consult a physician.

7. Accept changes as they occur. People with AD change and so do their needs. They often require care beyond what can be provided at home. A thorough investigation of available care options should make transitions easier along with support and assistance from those who care about the client and family.

8. Seek legal and financial planning. Consult an attorney and discuss issues related to durable power of attorney, living wills and trusts, future medical care, housing, and other key considerations. Planning now alleviates stress later. If possible and appropriate, involve the person with AD and other family members in planning activities and decisions.

9. Be realistic. Until a cure is found, the progression of AD is irreversible although the care provided does make a difference in the client's quality of life. Neither the caregiver nor the client with AD can control the circumstances and behaviors that will occur. Grieve for the losses experienced but focus on the positive moments as they occur and enjoy the good times.

10. Give credit, not guilt. Occasionally, the caregiver may lose patience and at times be unable to provide all of the care the way he or she would like. Give the person credit. Being a devoted caregiver is not something to feel guilty about.

The following are some practical suggestions for family and health caregivers:

- be knowledgeable about AD and the behaviors to expect
- talk about experiences and share feelings and stresses with others
- always ask for help when it is needed
- pace yourself and take frequent breaks
- plan physical activities to work off stress
- keep a sense of humor
- be realistic about the client

Nurses and HCAs should teach and follow the three "Es":

1. Encourage outside activities.
2. Expand your support group.
3. Educate yourself.

The impact on the caregiver of a family member with AD is usually expressed in the following ways:

1. Denial of the situation is a normal response but can be counterproductive if it encourages unrealistic expectations of the client's condition and prevents the more positive response of acceptance.
2. Feelings of anger, guilt, and resentment of the client, of other family members not helping enough, and the burden being too great. Even time away from the AD client can cause guilt.
3. Isolation, especially social, is real because the AD client often behaves in an unacceptable manner.
4. Depression is a natural response to feelings of lack of control over the illness or disease. Unexpressed anger and sadness in the caregiver may result in physical illness and depression.
5. Grief is a common response because of the loss of the loved one, physically and mentally.

It is essential for caregivers experiencing these feelings to express them freely. This can be done in a support group, with a professional counselor, or with a health caregiver who simply listens with care and concern. A medical social worker can be brought into the home to help counsel the family, if necessary. Figure 8–2 shows the medical social worker talking to the client.

HCAs who offer care to clients with AD all day every day can experience feeling similar to those of the family caregiver. It is very important for the employer to recognize signs of health caregiver burnout which is essentially the same as that of the family's. In-house support groups offer HCAs the same support the family gets from the outside. The HCA who recognizes signs

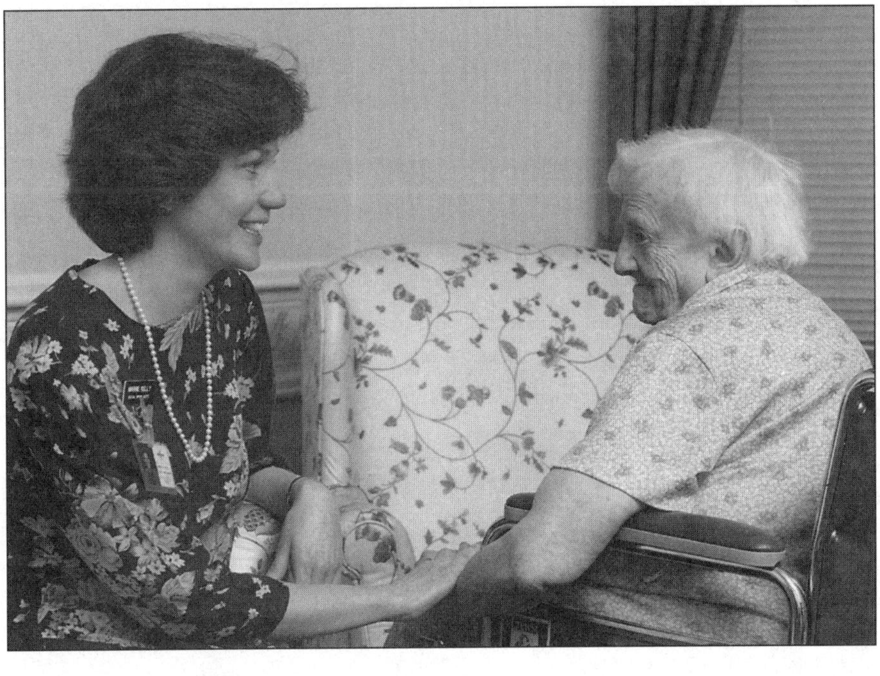

Figure 8–2 The social worker is concerned with the client's psychosocial needs.

of stress should go to the supervisor early and be honest about his or her feelings. Care of all caregivers is essential to the long-term care of AD clients.

BASIC TECHNIQUES FOR CARING FOR THE CLIENT WITH AD

technique a systematic approach or procecure to accomplish a task

A **technique** is a systematic approach or procedure to accomplish a difficult task. The basic techniques for HCAs working with dementia clients are described by the Alzheimer's Association and should be considered first before offering hands-on care. These include:

1. *Consistency*—The confused and disoriented individual functions better in a dependable environment. The person with dementia is upset by change and the already distorted sense of time is worsened by a change in schedule or if surroundings are unfamiliar.
2. *Calm*—The individual with dementia is especially sensitive to the moods and emotions of those around him or her. The HCA's calm approach, patience, and understanding creates an environment where the client feels safe and secure.
3. *Reassuring Gestures*—The confused individual can no longer depend on his or her own senses to assure a sense of well-being. The HCA must demonstrate verbally that the person is safe and being well cared for. The person with dementia is still able to understand feelings and emotions by means of nonverbal communication, even when he or she can no longer understand the spoken word. A touch or a smile increases the client's sense of security.
4. *Eye Contact*—The person suffering from dementia has great difficulty making sense of his or her environment. Frequent eye contact provides the client with some sense of stability and security.
5. *Voice Intonation*—The HCA's tone of voice and words are used to demonstrate respect for the client and acceptance of him or her. However, an angry or hostile tone adds to the client's confusion and fear.
6. *Simple Communication*—The HCA should communicate with the client by expressing one idea at a time. Simple sentences that require the interpretation of only one thought are easier for the client to remember and are easier to respond to.
7. *Distraction*—The best way to deal with inappropriate behavior is to identify the client's feelings and move on to another activity. Once distracted, the client will likely forget what was disturbing.

8. *Punctuality*—Keep the client's wait time for an appointment to a minimum. The client's confusion and disorientation will increase if he or she has to wait in an unfamiliar environment. The client may not understand, forget why he or she is waiting, become anxious, or wander off.

The HCA who specializes in caring for clients with AD is:

- able to handle stressful situations with a calm attitude
- more creative than the average person in handling clients
- willing to make a long-term commitment to the client and family
- reliable and able to accept responsibility
- empathetic to the client's fears, behaviors, and anxiety levels
- educated about the progression and degeneration of the disease
- caring, patient, and honest
- self-confident and secure about his or her self-esteem
- able to keep a sense or humor

PROBLEM BEHAVIORS OF THE CLIENT WITH AD AND APPROPRIATE RESPONSES

Problem behaviors are very common in the client with AD. Table 8–1 contains problem behaviors and possible solutions for each.

Table 8–1 Alzheimer's Disease Guidelines for Caregivers

Client	HHHA Actions/Responsibilities
Has difficulty communicating	• approach the client with a friendly facial expression • be calm • stand in front of the client • try to maintain eye contact: touch the client to attract attention or regain it • speak in a low, calm, reassuring tone of voice (if the client has a hearing problem, follow the instructions in the care plan) • speak slowly and give the client time to answer • if necessary, repeat the statement or question: do not change the wording. • keep the language simple and express only one idea at a time • lead the client in answering if he cannot find the right words; point to objects to provide cues • do not become impatient
Has difficulty walking	• provide a safe environment by removing scatter rug, not waxing floors, picking up and putting away objects the client may not see small footstools, doorstops, plants, pet toys, and dishes, and provide the client with chairs with arms for support • show the client what you want him or her to do and provide support • do not hurry the client • if the client is unsteady and is using an aid such as a cane or walker, do not let him or her out of your sight

(continues)

Table 8–1 continued	
Client	**HHHA Actions/Responsibilities**
	• be sure the client's shoes fit properly • always use proper body mechanics when helping the client • keep the client walking as long as possible (this becomes even more important as the disease progresses)
Experiences changes in eating patterns	• meals must be served at the same time each day • meals should look appetizing and be served at the proper temperature • give the client one course and one utensil at a time; do not give the client a choice of foods • if the client must be fed, do so slowly and cut the food into small pieces • nutritious snacks should be kept on hand • always encourage fluids • as the client loses the ability to chew, introduce soft foods; a blender can be used to liquify foods • as the client loses the ability to use utensils, serve finger foods • maintain the diet plan included in the overall care plan • weigh the client regularly (at least once weekly) and record the weight
Tends to wander	• be sure the client wears an ID bracelet or necklace • sew labels to each piece of clothing—labels should include the client's name, address, and telephone number • keep doors locked; make sure the bell or chimes are in working order • place large print signs on doors such as "Do not go out" or "Turn around" • if the client insists on going out, do not argue but go with him or her (lock the door and take the keys) • after a few minutes, suggest returning to the house to rest • try to distract the client from leaving by turning to another activity that the client enjoys (Alzheimer's clients often respond to music) • keep a recent photograph of the client at hand in the event the client does wander off and is not in the immediate neighborhood • if the client does leave unnoticed and you cannot find him or her, notify all family members, the police, and the agency
Experiences incontinence	• remember that the client cannot control this behavior • do not scold or punish the client • treat the client with respect • set up a regular schedule for toileting and follow it • encourage fluids as usual to prevent dehydration • mark the bathroom clearly with a large print sign and a picture • keep the client clean and dry; use simple washable clothing • recognize the client's verbal and nonverbal language • check the skin regularly for signs of irritation
Exhibits restlessness and agitation in late afternoon (sundown syndrome)	• decrease the level of activity in late afternoon to reduce potential stress • play soft, soothing music • do not try to reason the client out of this behavior; the client has no control over his or her actions • do not institute sudden changes into the routine which will confuse and upset the client • appointments and trips should be scheduled for morning and early afternoon • do not restrain or argue with the client • try to distract the client with quiet, simple activities • make sure the client has adequate exercise during the day

(continues)

THE CAREGIVER 103

Table 8–1 continued	
Client	**HHHA Actions/Responsibilities**
Experiences sleeping disturbances	• the client may exhibit less need for sleep • try to keep the client active during the day so he or she will feel the need for sleep • the client should drink caffeine-free beverages • establish a bedtime routine and follow it • make sure the client is toileted before going to bed • make sure there are no loud noises; soft music may help • the client may feel more secure with a nightlight • keep a nightlight on in the bathroom and keep the door open
Needs help with bathing and oral hygiene	• permit the client to do as much as he or she can; suggest steps if necessary • ensure the client's safety when bathing; use hand holds, nonslip mats, tub seats, and the like. • organize all the necessary equipment before you take the client to the bathroom • stay calm and pleasant; try to make it a pleasurable experience for the client • do not leave the client alone when bathing • schedule bathing when the client is least agitated • do not force the client to bathe; wait until he or she is calm and try again • give the client a sponge bath if all attempts to tub bathe or shower fail • cleanliness must be maintained; consult with your supervisor if the client continues to exhibit resistance to bathing • if the client cannot provide oral care, even with coaxing, brush his or her teeth yourself or clean the dentures
Experiences delusions, hallucinations, and inappropriate (catastrophic) reactions to normal events	• what the client sees or hears is real to him or her • do not argue or reason with the client • maintain a clam, ordered environment • reassure the client that you are there to protect him or her • if the client becomes violent, stay out of his or her way • if the client becomes agitated, try to distract him or her with an activity you know he or she likes; a small snack of a favorite food may work sufficiently to restore calm • if the client attacks you verbally, do not take it personally • the client may accuse you of stealing; again, do not take it personally
Exhibits improper sexual behavior	• remember that the client is confused and disoriented • do not overreact; remain calm • do not scold or argue with the client • do not try to reason with the client • if the client undresses, provide a robe or dress him or her • if the client is in public when inappropriate behavior takes place, distract the client and remove him or her from the scene • plan ahead ways in which you can distract the client • provide appropriate touching to show that you care for and value the client

Most of the behavior of the client with AD is inappropriate. However, when the client exhibits an appropriate behavior, the caregiver or HCA should praise this positive behavior to reinforce it. It is important to keep in mind that the client has no control

> **Helpful Hints:** A simple smile or saying "that was very good" encourages better behavior in clients with AD.

over his or her behavior, usually does not remember the behavior, and shows no remorse for causing disruptions or problems.

There are additional behaviors of AD and other dementia conditions that the HCA should understand and consider before hands-on care begins. These are listed below with suggestions for appropriate HCA responses that promote a more cooperative relationship between the client and the HCA.

Behavior	Appropriate Response
Agitated or combative	Try to determine the trigger for the behavior and stop it. Use a calm, slow voice and avoid restraints.
Depression	Report to the supervisor. Encourage activity and listen with concern. Encourage independent behavior.
Suspicion and/or paranoia	Do not argue or disagree. Realize there is a loss of judgment. Show respect and foster trust by going about tasks in a caring manner.
Confusion and/or disorientation	Use client's name and your name frequently and say where you are. Reassure the client that he or she is safe.
Hiding things or stealing	Lock the closets and cupboards and keep an extra set of keys. Do not argue about items that are missing. Do not accuse or confront the client.
Sexual behavior	Realize the client has lost the sense of right or wrong. Use distractions and remove the client from the situation. Remind the client of the appropriate behavior.
Pacing or restlessness	Remind the client of where he or she is and reassure him or her that someone is staying nearby. Provide a calm environment with familiar surrounds. Try distractions such as playing music or turning on the television. Exercise may help. Do not interfere or restrain the client.
Wandering	If caused by boredom, keep the client busy. Nighttime wandering is less if there are no naps during the day.
Delusions and/or hallucinations	Respond by reassuring the client that he or she is safe. Be calm and use distractions.
Violent actions	This behavior is usually short-term and not directed at anyone person-

Catastrophic reactions (overreaction to a situation, combativeness, shouting, anger, irritability, sudden changes in mood)

ally. Protect yourself. Move away and stay calm. Get help and report the behavior to the supervisor. Observe for triggers and events causing the behavior. Provide a quiet place for the client. Back off on tasks and demands. Do not ask questions until the client calms down. Determine if the client is experiencing pain or discomfort.

Possible triggers of severe reactions include:
- overstimulation
- fatigue
- change of routine
- change of caregiver
- too many choices or questions
- hunger
- pain or discomfort
- need for toileting
- too much noise
- too much activity
- too difficult a task
- scolding
- insecurity
- feeling rushed

Helpful Hints: The HCA should teach the family to lower these stimuli in situations when caring for a client with AD

CARING TECHNIQUES

There are specialized techniques that apply in the care of a person who has Alzheimer's. Some of these are contrary to the way we were taught to treat others.

1. Join in the client's make-believe world or life in the past. The person with Alzheimer's is often not able to live in the present and feels safer and more comfortable living in the past as he or she remembers it now.

2. Do not accuse persons with Alzheimer's of lying. Their understanding of the world is different from yours. In order to make their world logical, they often fill in gaps of memory with past experiences instead of with what is actually happening. Relate to the underlying feeling of fear or loss of security rather than give a specific statement of accusation.

3. Use distractions. A temporary change of subject often solves the problem and takes the person's attention away from the

undesirable behavior. The person's forgetfulness can work in the caregiver's favor.

4. Do not be upset if the person makes unkind remarks or is not tactful. A confused person often misjudges situations and is overly suspicious. Remember that the person has lost the memory of good manners.
5. Follow a simple, set routine. Eliminate distracting noises and activities if possible. Change is upsetting to the client with AD.
6. Encourage the person to perform as many activities unassisted as his or her abilities allow. For example, the person may be able to dress alone if the clothes are laid out in the right order or held so they can be slipped on. Figure 8–3 shows the HCA assisting the client in selecting her own clothes.
7. Demonstrate appropriate actions by modeling correct methods. For example, move arm up and down to simulate brushing teeth.

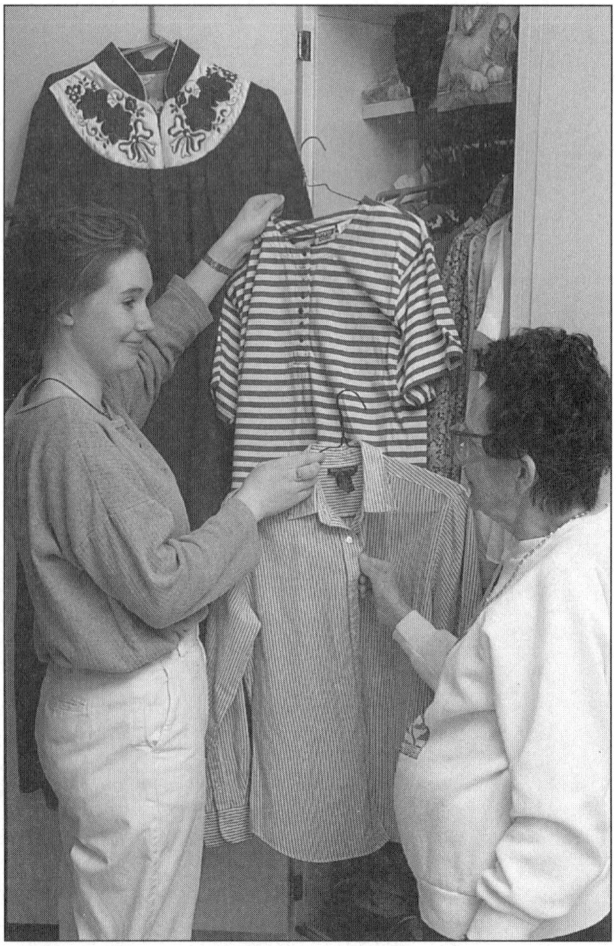

Figure 8–3 The HCA is assisting the client to select clothes to wear.

8. Praise actions as often as possible.
9. Create a safe environment. Remove all hazards that could be dangerous to the client.
10. Avoid situations that bring about frustration and anger. Try to anticipate problems and prevent them from happening.
11. Help the person get adequate exercise. This is an important part of the daily routine.
12. Be aware that the person with Alzheimer's has lost the ability to keep track of time which causes anxiety and frustration. A person feels deserted when only a few minutes have elapsed. Reassure the client as much as possible.
13. Do not assume that the person understands and acts on messages, either written or verbal.
14. Break each activity into small steps. Encourage the person to take each task one step at a time and talk through each step.
15. Encourage clients to participate in activities which are pleasurable to them. Be aware that they may have short spans of attention. Find out what activities they have enjoyed in the past and continue to find rewarding.
16. Remember that the person may have lost the ability to judge between safe and unsafe conditions. Evaluate each situation and do not let the person wander into a potentially dangerous situation.

All humans have certain levels of basic needs which must be met (see Figure 8–4). The first level of basic physical needs include food, water, and oxygen. The second level contains safety and protection. If a person does not feel safe, this need overtakes him or her. The client with AD lives in a paranoid state of mind in which he or she does not feels safe. The HCA and the caregiver should assure the client that he or she is safe at all times.

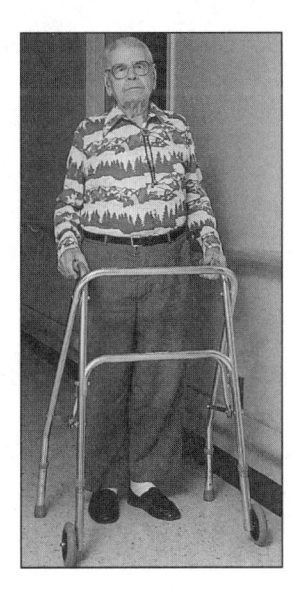

Figure 8–4 People meet needs in order of priority of importance. Physical needs must be satisfied first.

Other needs on this level relate to structure and order. This is especially important for the client with AD. Any change in the usual structure of the client's life leads to confusion and anger. It is important to maintain a routine as much as possible.

The final level of this hierarchy comprises psychosocial needs. The caregiver and family should focus on fulfilling these needs for themselves because often the family's needs are forgotten when caring for a client with AD.

REVIEW QUESTIONS

1. Caring for most clients with AD is a _____ hour-a-day task.
2. The term _____ usually refers to that person who is primarily responsible for caring for the client from day to day.
3. _____% of all caregivers are women.
4. Four basic rules for any person caring for a client with AD are:
    a. Keep _____
    b. Respond by _____
    c. Remain _____
    d. Constantly _____
5. There are _____ levels in Maslow's hierarchy of needs.
6. Which of the following is not a stress management technique?
    a. listening to music
    b. deep breathing
    c. passive progressive relaxation
    d. sleeping
    e. bio-feedback
7. Which of the following are tension relievers?
    a. visualization
    b. curling toes
    c. yawning
    d. massages
    e. all of the above
8. True or False? The Alzheimer's Association states that getting a diagnosis and knowing resources can reduce caregiver stress.
9. True or False? Delegating tasks is not a tension reliever.
10. True or False? Denial of a situation can have a great impact on a family caring for a client with AD.
11. True or False? Grief can be a common response to the loss of a loved one even before death occurs.
12. Unscramble the following key term from the chapter: rraeciveg _____

CHAPTER 9

Safety and Emergencies

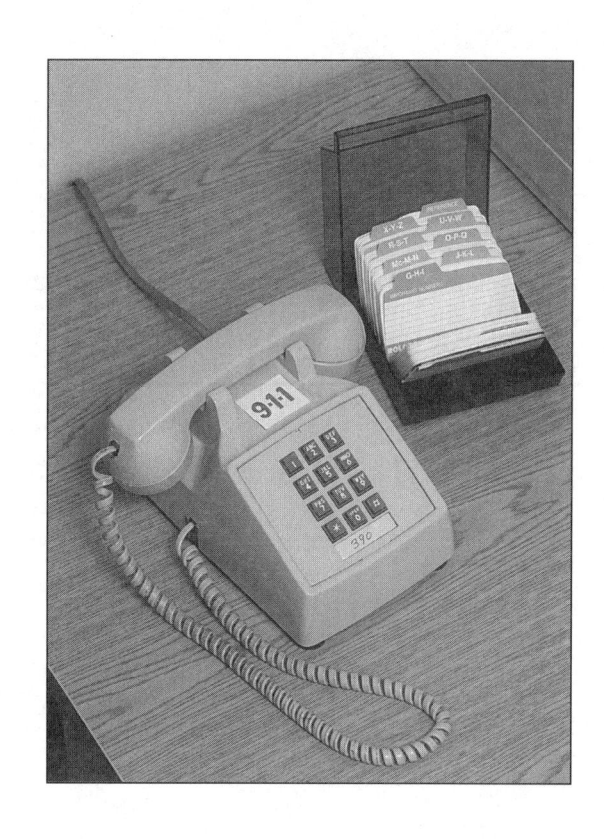

OBJECTIVES

Upon reading this chapter and completing the review questions, the home care aide should be able to:
1. Have a greater understanding of safety and emergency situations.
2. Observe the environment of the client in terms of safety measures.
3. Name the most common safety hazards in the home.
4. List some conditions that promote safety and prevent falls.
5. State some basic facts of medication safety.
6. Be familiar with emergency measures in home care.
7. Demonstrate an understanding of positioning the client and transfer safety.

KEY TERMS

aseptic	pathogens
confused	personal protective equipment (PPE)
disoriented	prevention
flammable	safe environment
infection	standard precautions

INTRODUCTION

The home can be an unsafe area for the homebound client as well as for the HCA who cares for that client. Clients who are ill and weak are more prone to accidents at home and are usually unable to handle an emergency.

Safety is one of the HCA's responsibilities. He or she can create a **safe environment** for the client by preventing, correcting, or eliminating conditions that could cause accidents and assisting the client and family in taking measures to be prepared for crisis intervention. **Prevention** is a means to slow or stop the number of accidents in the home.

All clients cared for in the home have the right to a healthy and safe environment. When caring for the client with AD who has poor judgment or is unsteady, the hazards are greater. Therefore, the responsibilities for client safety are increased and the caregiver becomes the person who truly safeguards the client. The nurse on the case should assess the home for safety carefully because the potential for injury to these persons is greater than the average client.

Falls are the leading cause of death or injury in persons over the age of sixty-five. The person with AD who falls and injures himself or herself becomes an even greater nursing challenge because all of the caring problems are present but are multiplied by the symptoms of the disease process of AD.

safe environment an environment in which a person has a very low risk of illness or injury

prevention to slow or stop a potentially hazardous situation

Helpful Hints: It is the HCA's responsibility to observe the home in related to the client's safety on every visit.

OBSERVING FOR POTENTIAL RISKS

The potential for injury is especially high in clients with AD. When observing for potential risks, the HCA should consider the following:

- the client's level of functioning
- the client's emotional state
- incontinence
- the use of medications
- poor eyesight
- poor hearing
- balance problems
- history of alcohol and/or substance abuse

The HCA is responsible for keeping the home environment safe and free from hazards. The client has very little regard for his or her own safety and it is important to review some of the basic safety rules and apply them to the situation when caring for a client with AD. Some general safety measures for clients in the home are:

- smoking should not be allowed unless someone is with the client every minute; matches should be locked up
- electrical cords should be off the floor and out of sight
- loose rugs should be removed
- stairs, halls, and doorways should be kept free of clutter
- furniture should be arranged to allow free movement because clients with AD walk constantly
- grab bars should be installed in the bathtub, shower, and by the toilet
- nonskid rubber mats should be placed in the bathtub and shower
- a first-aid kit should be kept in the home at all times
- smoke alarms and fire extinguishers should be in the home at all times
- all medicine should be locked away
- the shoes worn by the client should have nonskid soles
- all hazardous tools and firearms should be locked away
- emergency numbers should be close to the telephone, especially 911. The HCA should discuss emergency communications with the family and report to the supervisor if problems exist (see Figure 9–1)

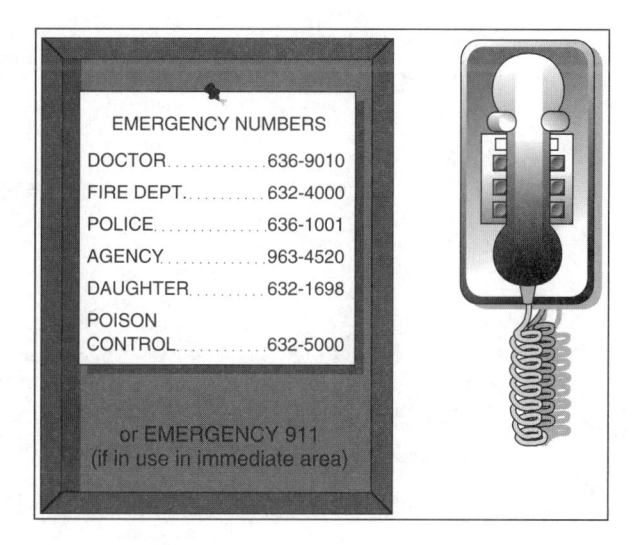

Figure 9–1 Important phone numbers posted next to the phone may save precious moments at the time of an emergency.

EMERGENCY NUMBERS
DOCTOR............636-9010
FIRE DEPT..........632-4000
POLICE.............636-1001
AGENCY............963-4520
DAUGHTER.........632-1698
POISON CONTROL...632-5000

or EMERGENCY 911
(if in use in immediate area)

- night lights should be provided everywhere in the home
- the temperature of the hot water heater should be lowered to prevent problems when there is no one else around
- poison should be locked away

The bathroom can be a potentially hazardous area and the following should be considered:

- the toilet seat should be secure and guard rails placed at the toilet
- the client should be able to get up and down safely
- hot and cold water faucets should be correctly marked
- floors should never remain wet and slippery
- night lights should be installed in bathrooms

The kitchen area also can be especially dangerous for clients with AD. The following safety guidelines are specific for the kitchen area:

- the kitchen should have a fire extinguisher and a smoke alarm
- the handles of pans should be turned toward the back of the stove when in use
- the HCA should observe the client when he or she is using the stove (see Figure 9–2)

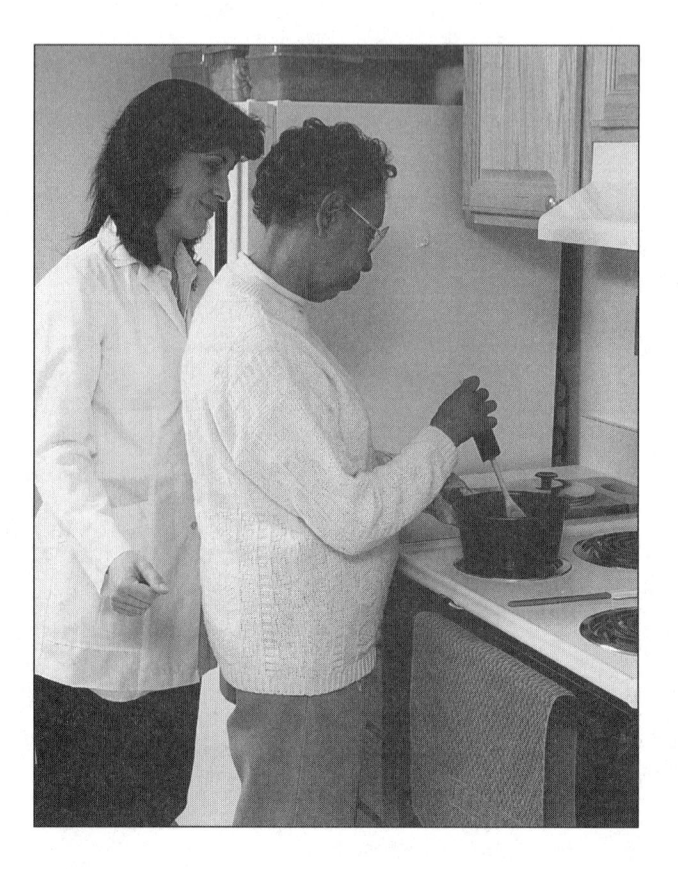

Figure 9–2 Always supervise the client when she is using the stove.

- grease and liquids should be thoroughly cleaned when spilled especially on the floor
- cleaning liquids such as polishes, bleaches, and detergents should be kept locked away
- nonbreakable dishes are recommended
- sharp knives should be kept in a locked drawer
- an escape plan should be created and posted in the kitchen with an exit route established before hand

The HCA should observe the home for safety at every visit. A safety checklist should be kept on the client's record and a weekly review done by the nurse and/or the HCA. The safety recommendations should be placed in a prominent place so that all family members and caregivers can refer to it easily and quickly.

MAINTAINING A SAFE ENVIRONMENT IN THE HOME

When the patient is admitted to home health care, the skilled nurse does a safety assessment of the home during the admission process. A safety checklist is usually included in the admission packet because safety measures and interventions begin at that time. The HCA follows up on this process and the nurse includes the client's family and the rest of the health care team when setting safety goals and determining if the goals have been met. The HCA should constantly assess the quality of the environment and look for safety hazards. If any are discovered, the HCA should report them to the supervisor immediately.

Helpful Hints: The HCA should correct a hazardous situation immediately such as clearing a cluttered stairway.

Helpful Hints: The agency is responsible for the client's safety. Therefore, the HCA as the agency's representative is also responsible for the client's safety.

A safe environment is one in which a person has a very low risk of illness or injury. Some elderly and frail persons cannot assume the responsibility of their own safety. Poor vision may play a part in a client's inability to be safe at home. This leads to falls, tripping, and misreading labels. Hearing loss is another factor affecting the client's safety as warning signals such as fire detectors may or may not be heard.

The most common safety hazards in the home are:
- damaged electrical wiring on large and small appliances
- faulty or uneven stairs
- loose rugs that slip and slide
- poisons
- **flammable** cleaning rags, mops, and brooms
- sharp objects such as knives, razors, and lawn tools
- wet floors
- cluttered hallways
- unstable furniture

flammable able to catch fire

114 CHAPTER 9

Figure 9-3 shows a stairway that is cluttered and Figure 9-4 shows damaged plugs and too many plugs in one outlet.

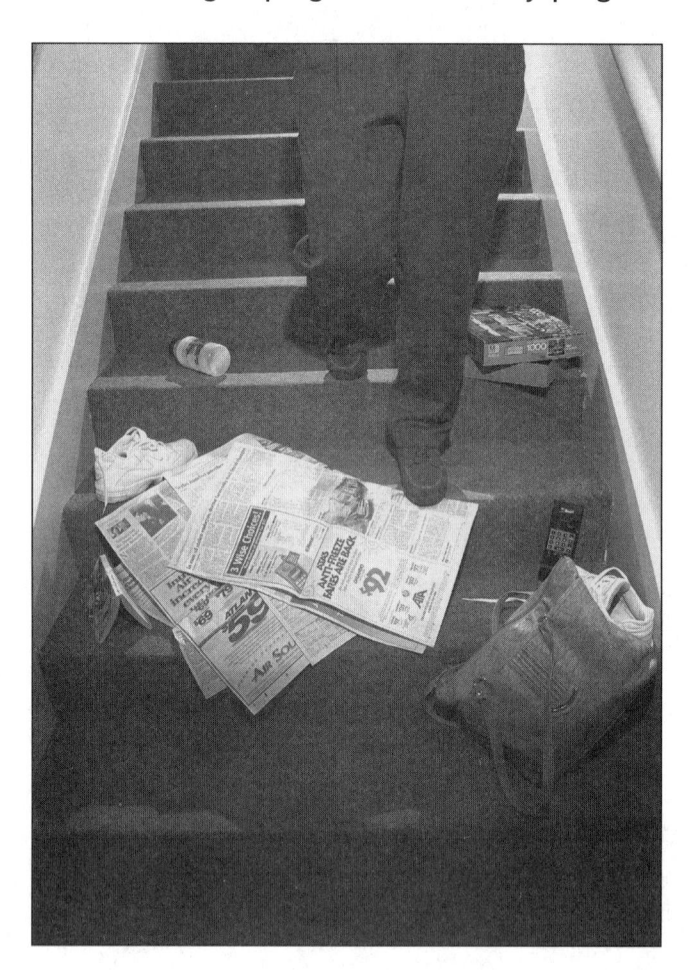

Figure 9-3 Cluttered stairway can be hazardous for the elderly client who has vision or balance problems.

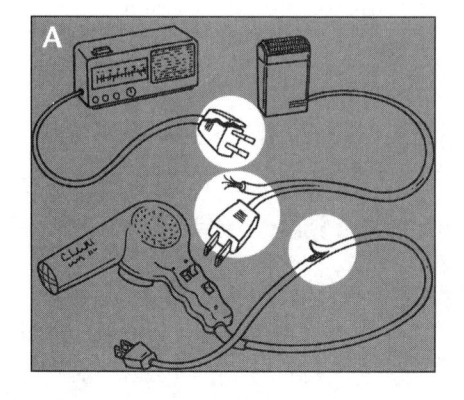

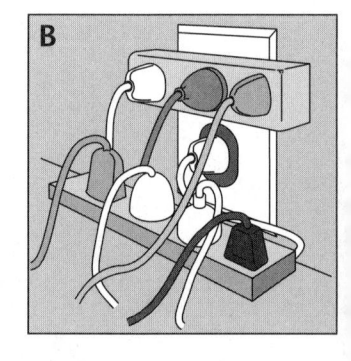

Figure 9-4 A. Cords in unsafe conditions. B. There are too many cords in this outlet

Falls

Falls are the most common accidents in the home, particularly among the elderly. Most falls occur in the bedroom or bathroom and are caused by slippery floors, throw rugs, poor lighting, cluttered floors, furniture that is out of place, or slippery bathtubs and showers. Some conditions that promote safety and prevent falls are:

1. Adequate lighting rooms and hallways.
2. Hand rails on both sides of stairs, in halls, and in bathrooms.
3. Carpeting tacked down and throw rugs avoided.
4. Nonskid shoes and slippers worn by clients when ambulating.
5. Nonskid waxes used on hardwood, tiled, or linoleum floors.
6. Floors uncluttered with toys and other objects.
7. Electrical cords and extension cords kept out of the path of the client.
8. Furniture left in place and not rearranged.
9. A telephone and lamp placed at the bedside.
10. Nonskid bathmats in tubs and showers.
11. Assistance for weak clients when they are walking, getting out of bed, getting out of the tub or shower, and with other activities ordered by the physician.
12. Call bell within easy reach.
13. Cracked steps, loose hand rails, and frayed carpets reported and repaired promptly.
14. Frequently used items placed within the client's easy reach.
15. The client's bed in the low position, except when bedside care is being given to minimize the distance from the bed to the floor.
16. Night lights in the client's room and hallways.
17. Floors kept free of spills and excess furniture.
18. Crutches, canes, and walkers fitted with nonskid tips.
19. Wheels on beds and wheelchairs locked when transferring clients to or from them.
20. Gates at the tops and bottoms of stairs when there are infants and toddlers in the home. The child should not be able to put his or her head through the gate bars.
21. Side rails installed on the client's bed if possible to prevent the client from falling out of bed.

Figure 9–5 shows safety bars for the bathtub.

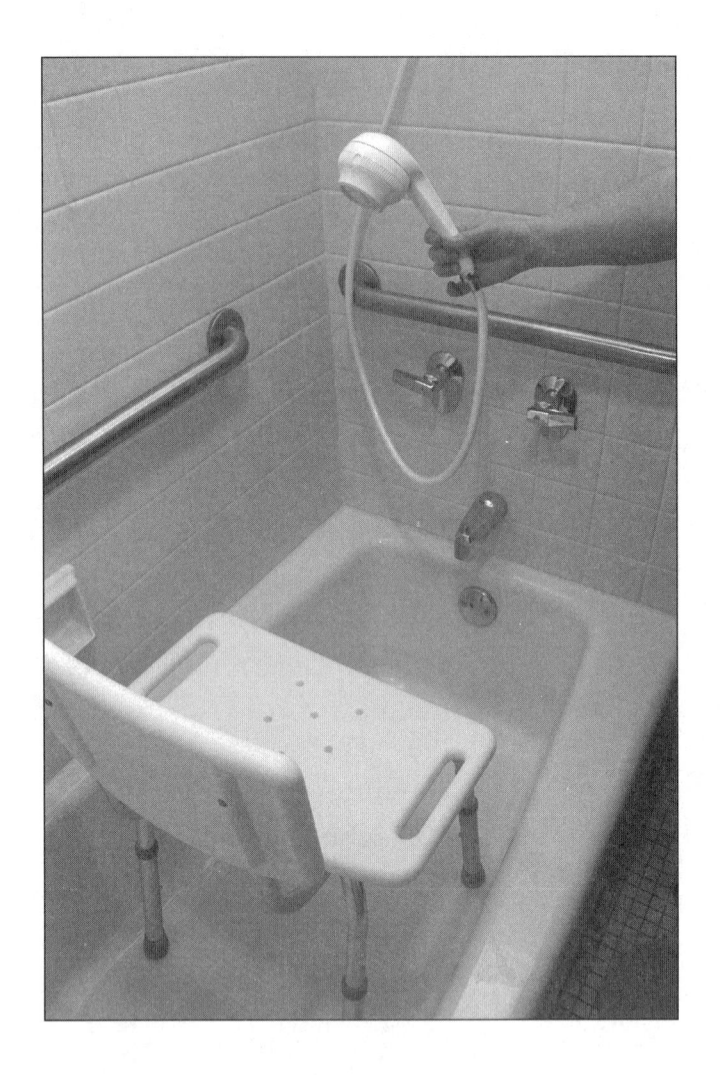

Figure 9-5 Safety features for the tub may include several types of bars and nonskid strips to allow the client to get into and out of the tub safely.

Helpful Hints: Keep your eyes and ears open for over-the-counter medication use and misuse that should be reported to the nurse and/or supervisor.

Medication Safety

Storage and disposal of medications in the home are major problem areas for home health workers. HCAs should never dispense or administer medication. However, the HCA needs information about certain medications because many clients receiving home care services are taking them. HCAs often hand medications to their clients, remind clients to take medications, and report their use, misuse, and effects to their supervisors. The client with AD is at high risk of taking medications that belong to other family members.

Some safety guidelines for medications are:

1. When cleaning the medicine cabinet, special care should be taken not to disturb medication container labels.
2. Medication containers should be replaced in the same position in the medicine cabinet after cleaning, because often clients expect a bottle to be in one position and do not look at the label.
3. If more than one person in the household is taking medications, keep the medications in separate rooms to avoid a client from taking the wrong medication.

4. Encourage the client to dispose of old medications correctly by flushing them down the toilet. Report the disposal to the supervisor.
5. The client should store medications in a specific area and tell the family members where it is. The medications should not be moved.
6. Know if there are special instructions for storage of medications such as refrigeration.
7. Never refer to medications as "candy."

The "five rights" for safely taking medications are:
1. The *right* client.
2. The *right* medication.
3. The *right* time.
4. The *right* way to take the medication (oral, and so forth).
5. The *right* dose.

EMERGENCY MEASURES IN HOME CARE

Helpful Hints: All HCAs should keep current on CPR and emergency measures.

HCAs may be called on to handle emergency situations in the home. All HCAs should have a basic first-aid course and a current basic life support course. Figure 9–6 shows first-aid procedures in case of a fire.

First Aid—What to Do
If you catch on fire:
DO NOT PANIC, DO NOT RUN—RUNNING WIll INCREASE THE FLAMES. Instead: 1. Stop 2. Drop to the ground 3. Roll. Continue to roll until you have completely put out the fire. 4. Remove clothing from affected area. Do not attempt to remove clothing that sticks. 5. Flush area with cool water. 6. Cover with a sterile pad or a clean sheet. 7. Seek immediate medical attention
If the burn is from a chemical:
1. Follow steps 4–7 and be sure to flush with cool water for 20–30 minutes. 2. If the eyes are involved, flush the eyes for at least 20 minutes or until medical attention arrives. 3. Remove contact lenses.
If the burn is electrical:
1. Turn off electrical source before touching victim. 2. Check for breathing and pulse. If absent, start Cardiopulmonary Resuscitation (CPR), if qualified. 3. Follow steps 4–7.

Figure 9–6 First aid—what to do.

Emergency Plans

Each emergency situation is different but the following general rules apply to any kind of emergency:

1. HCAs should know their limitations and not try a procedure that is unfamiliar.
2. HCAs should remain calm at all times. Being calm helps the client feel more secure.
3. HCAs should observe the client for life-threatening problems and should always check for breathing, pulse, and bleeding.
4. HCAs should keep the victim lying down or in the position which he or she was found. Never move the victim. Moving a victim could make the injury worse.
5. HCAs should perform necessary emergency measures.
6. HCAs should call for help or instruct someone to call 911. An operator will send emergency vehicles and personnel to the scene. The person calling 911 should give the following information to the operator:
   - the location including the street address and city or town
   - the phone number where the victim is located
   - what happened (a fall, choking) since fire equipment, police, and ambulances may be needed
   - how many people require emergency medical attention
   - the condition(s) of the victim(s,) any obvious injuries, and if there is a life-threatening situation
   - what aid is currently being given
7. HCAs should not remove the victim's clothing unless absolutely necessary.
8. The victim should be kept warm. Aides can cover the victim with a blanket or a coat.
9. HCAs should reassure the conscious victim by explaining what is happening and that help is on the way.
10. HCAs should not give the victim any foods or fluids.
11. HCAs should keep onlookers away from the victim to maintain his or her privacy.

Every home should have a plan in case of emergencies. The home with a client with AD or an elderly, frail, ill, or impaired person must take extra measures to plan ahead for emergency situations.

Figure 9-7 shows a HCA teaching the family the escape plan in case of fire.

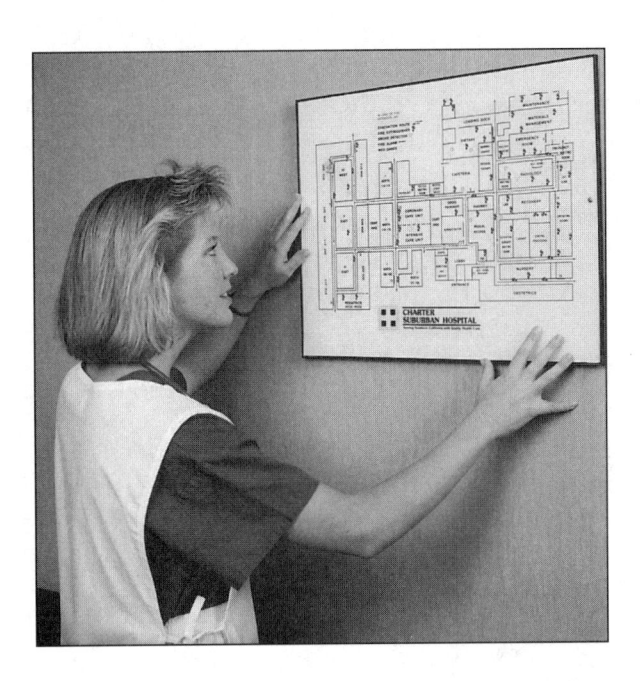

Figure 9–7 Client and family should know the escape plan in the event of a fire.

Reporting an accident or emergency by telephone should be done in a calm manner. It is important to have emergency numbers written next to the telephone(s). This list should include:

- Emergency Medical Services (EMS) (often 911) if available
- Police department
- Fire department
- Responsible family member at work
- The home care supervisor and agency
- Client's physician
- Nearest hospital
- Ambulance service (if different from EMS)
- Poison control center

If there is no telephone in the client's home, arrange in advance to use a neighbor's phone in case of an emergency.

Fire Safety

There are three major causes of fires in this country: faulty electrical equipment and wiring, overloaded electrical circuits, and smoking. Fire safety measures include:

1. Following the fire safety precautions in the use of oxygen.
2. Being sure all ashes, cigars, and cigarette butts are out before emptying ashtrays.
3. Providing ashtrays to clients who are allowed to smoke.
4. Emptying ashtrays into a metal container partly filled with sand or water. Do not empty ashtrays into wastebaskets or plastic containers lined with paper or plastic bags.

confused uncertain or unclear mentally

disoriented confusion in a sense of identity or location

5. Supervising smoking clients who cannot protect themselves. This includes **confused, disoriented**, and sedated clients. Never allow the client to smoke in bed.
6. Following the safety practices for using electrical equipment.
7. Supervising the play of children and keeping matches out of their reach.

Figure 9–8 shows the elements for combustion.

The following guidelines will help the HCA to protect the client if there is a fire. The HCA should:

- call the fire department
- have fire emergency numbers near the client's telephones
- plan escape routes from each room
- know where fire extinguishers are and how to use them
- know where fire alarms boxes are located
- turn off any oxygen or electrical equipment in the general area of the fire
- get the client and others out of the house
- leave right away if the fire gets out of control
- close door if the home is vacated
- crawl, keeping heads close to the floor if the area is filled with smoke
- cover faces with a damp cloth or towel in a smoke-filled area
- feel any doors before they are opened; do not open a door that feels hot or if smoke is coming from around the door
- open a cool door slowly, keeping the head to the side (doors should be closed immediately if smoke or heat rushes in)
- stuff blankets, clothes, towels, linens, coats, or other cloth at the bottom of the door if the client is trapped inside.
- open a window for air and hang a piece of cloth outside the window to attract attention

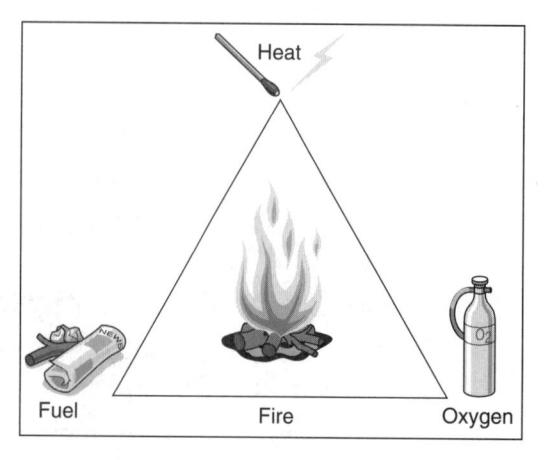

Figure 9–8 The fire triangle—elements needed for combustion (burning)

SAFETY AND EMERGENCIES **121**

The HCA should be able to use a fire extinguisher (see Figure 9–9). Local fire departments often give demonstrations on how to operate them. Some agencies require all employees to demonstrate how to use a fire extinguisher.

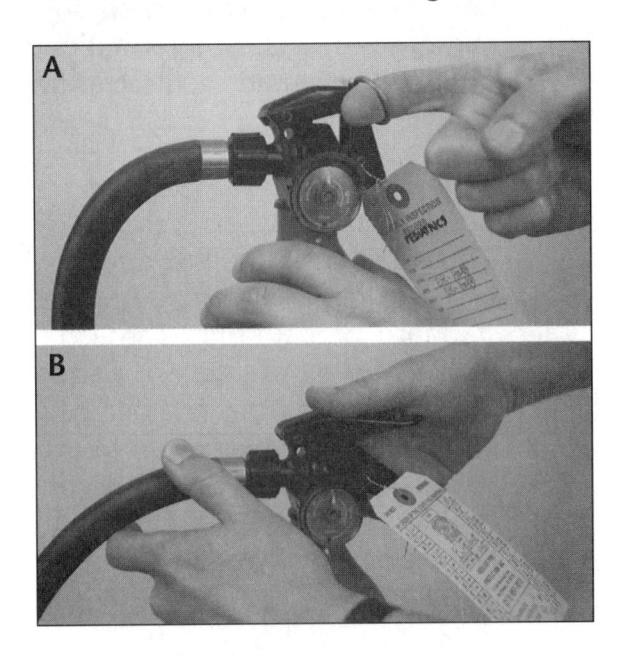

Figure 9–9 Use of the fire extinguisher. A. Remove pin. B. Push top handle down.

Figure 9–10 shows the HCA protecting the client when escaping a fire.

Helpful Hints: Do not forget that the escape of a disabled or elderly client is slower than that of others.

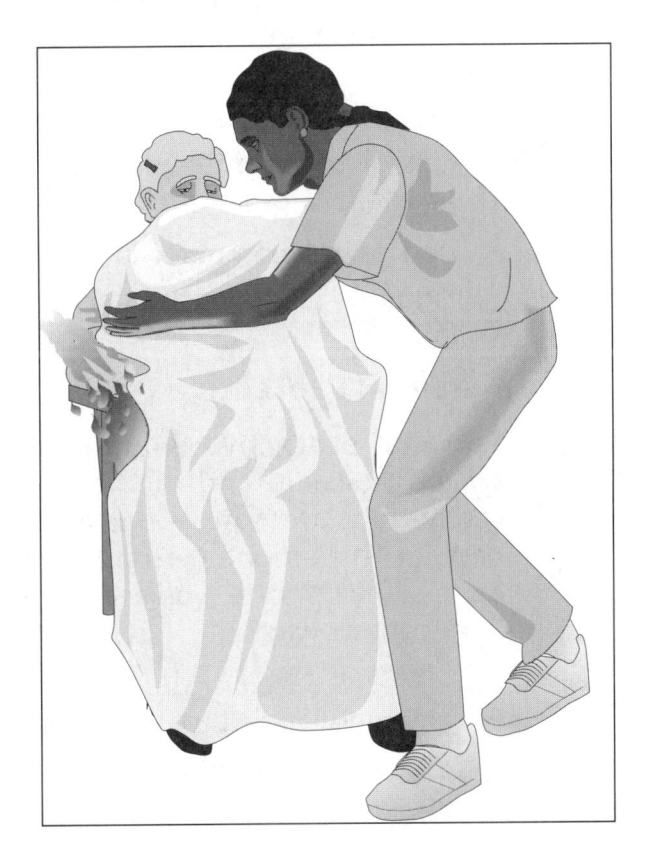

Figure 9–10 The HCA is protecting the client while trying to extinguish the fire.

INFECTION CONTROL

All home health personnel must be careful to use proper measures to control infection. The client with AD is at no greater or lesser risk for **infection** than any other client. HCAs should keep current on the latest information to protect the client, the family, other workers, and themselves from infection.

infection germs enter the body and cause disease

Universal Precautions

Universal precautions were developed in 1985 by the Centers for Disease Control and Prevention (CDC). These guidelines were adhered to until they were updated in 1996. They are now called standard precautions. These guidelines apply to all healthcare workers for all clients, no matter what the diagnosis or for what illness or injury they are being treated. If proper precautions are not taken, **pathogens** can be transmitted by the HCAs to themselves, their families, other clients, and their families by means of contamination on skin and clothing. Universal precautions protect against many different types of infections including AIDS, tuberculosis (TB), and Hepatitis B.

pathogen disease-causing microorganisms

Standard Precautions

The Centers for Disease Control and Prevention published new recommendations in 1996 called **standard precautions**. This new information is based on several years of research and data collection to:

- improve the criteria for universal precautions
- change some of the medical terminology
- offer new information on drug resistant pathogens
- update isolation guidelines

Figure 9–11 shows the standard precautions

standard precautions guidelines published by the CDC to prevent the spread of pathogens

Personal Protective Equipment

Personal protective equipment (PPE) provides a barrier between the client and the health care worker. When used correctly, PPE provides a barrier that prevents the transfer of pathogens from one person to another. Standard precautions require all health care workers to wear PPE anytime they expect to have contact with:

1. blood
2. any moist body fluid except sweat, secretions, or excretions
3. mucous membranes
4. nonintact skin

personal protective equipment (PPE) provides a barrier between the client and the health care worker. When used correctly, PPE provides a barrier that prevents the transfer of pathogens from one person to the other.

STANDARD PRECAUTIONS FOR INFECTION CONTROL

Wash Hands (Plain soap)
Wash after touching blood, body fluids, secretions, excretions, and contaminated items. Wash immediately after gloves are removed and between patient contacts. Avoid transfer of microorganisms to other patients or environments.

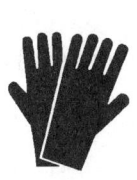

Wear Gloves
Wear when touching blood, body fluids, secretions, excretions, and contaminated items. Put on clean gloves just before touching mucous membranes and nonintact skin. Change gloves between tasks and procedures on the same patient after contact with material that may contain high concentrations of microorganisms. Remove gloves promptly after use, before touching noncontaminated items and environmental surfaces, and before going to another patient, and wash hands immediately to avoid transfer of microorganisms to other patients or environments.

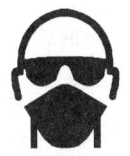

Wear Mask and Eye Protection or Face Shield
Protect mucous membranes of the eyes, nose and mouth during procedures and patient-care activities that are likely to generate splashes or sprays of blood, body fluids, secretions, or excretions.

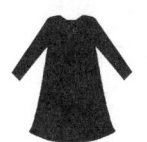

Wear Gown
Protect skin and prevent soiling of clothing during procedures that are likely to generate splashes or sprays of blood, body fluids, secretions, or excretions. Remove a soiled gown as promptly as possible and wash hands to avoid transfer of microorganisms to other patients or environments.

Patient-Care Equipment
Handle used patient-care equipment soiled with blood, body fluids, secretions, or excretions in a manner that prevents skin and mucous membrane exposures, contamination of clothing, and transfer of microorganisms to other patients and environments. Ensure that reusable equipment is not used for the care of another patient until it has been appropriately cleaned and reprocessed and single use items are properly discarded.

Environmental Control
Follow hospital procedures for routine care, cleaning, and disinfection of environmental surfaces, beds, bedrails, bedside equipment and other frequently touched surfaces.

Linen
Handle, transport, and process used linen soiled with blood, body fluids, secretions, or excretions in a manner that prevents exposure and contamination of clothing, and avoids transfer of microorganisms to other patients and environments.

Occupational Health and Bloodborne Pathogens
Prevent injuries when using needles, scalpels, and other sharp instruments or devices; when handling sharp instruments after procedures; when cleaning used instruments; and when disposing of used needles.

Never recap used needles using both hands or any other technique that involves directing the point of a needle towards any part of the body; rather, use either a one-handed "scoop" technique or a mechanical device designed for holding the needle sheath.

Do not remove used needles from disposable syringes by hand, and do not bend, break, or otherwise manipulate used needles by hand. Place used disposable syringes and needles, scalpels, blades, and other sharp items in puncture-resistant sharps containers located as close as practical to the area in which the items were used, and place reusable syringes and needles in a puncture-resistant container for transport to the reprocessing area.

Use resuscitation devices as an alternative to mouth-to-mouth resuscitation.

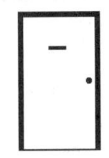

Patient Placement
Use a private room for a patient who contaminates the environment or who does not (or cannot be expected to) assist in maintaining appropriate hygiene or environmental control. Consult Infection Control if a private room is not available.

Figure 9–11 Standard precautions (Courtesy of BREVIS Corporation, Salt Lake City, UT)

PPE includes gloves, water resistant gowns, face shields, masks and goggles. HCAs should follow the agency's policies for use of PPE in routine tasks.

Some new medical terms associated with infection control include:

Visible—able to be seen with the eye

Body Substance Isolation—precautions requiring special handling of all fluids

Drug Resistant—disease-causing organisms that resist treatment with normal antibiotics

Reservoir—a human being who has an infection that can be spread to others

Airborne Transmission—tiny microbes that spread disease in the air over long distances such as TB.

Contact Transmission—tiny microbes spread through direct contact with body fluids such as urine.

Droplet Transmission—disease spread by respiratory secretions or droplets in the air within a distance of three feet.

Transmission-Based Precautions—CDC recommendations for isolating clients with certain diseases in addition to the standard precautions (Figure 9-12).

Higher-Efficiency Particulate Air Mask (HEPA)—a special mask with tiny pores to prevent airborne transmissions.

Table 9-1 Diseases requiring transmission-based isolation precautions.

Disease or Condition	Type of Precautions
AIDS	Standard (or reverse if facility policy)
Chickenpox	Airborne and Contact
Diarrhea	Standard
Drug resistant skin infections	Contact
German measles	Droplet
Head or body lice	Contact
Hepatitis, type A	Standard. Use contact if diarrhea or incontinent patient
Hepatitis, other types	Standard
HIV disease	Standard
Impetigo	Contact
Infected pressure sore with no drainage	Standard
Infected pressure sore with heavy drainage	Contact
Infectious diarrhea caused by a known pathogen	Contact
Measles	Airborne
Mumps	Droplet
Oral or genital herpes	Standard
Scabies	Contact
Syphilis	Standard
Tuberculosis of the lungs	Airborne
Widespread shingles	Airborne and contact

Use standard precautions in addition to other types of precautions listed.

Pathogens, which are the cause of infections, can be controlled with good cleaning techniques and maintenance. It is important to keep an **aseptic** environment for the client. Some common aseptic practices include:

- washing hands before and after touching the client
- washing hands after urinating, having a bowel movement, or changing tampons or sanitary napkins
- washing hands before handling or preparing food
- washing fruits and vegetables before serving them

aseptic absence of pathogens

- encouraging each family member to use his or her own towels, washcloths, toothbrush, drinking glass, and other personal care items
- using disposable cups and dishes for clients with an infection
- encouraging the client to cover the nose and mouth with tissues when coughing, sneezing, or blowing his or her nose
- making sure there is a plastic or paper bag for used tissues
- practicing good personal hygiene
- bathing, washing hair, and brushing teeth regularly
- encouraging clients to wash their hands often, especially after toileting and before eating
- washing cooking and eating utensils with soap and water after they have been used
- cleaning cooking and eating surfaces with soap and water or a disinfectant
- not leaving food sitting out and uncovered, closing all food containers, and refrigerating foods that could spoil
- not using food that smells bad or looks discolored
- checking the expiration date on food (do not use it if the date has passed)
- changing water in flower vases daily
- removing dead plants and flowers from the home
- dusting furniture with a damp cloth and using a damp mop for floors (this helps prevent the movement of dust in the air)
- emptying garbage daily using large, sturdy plastic bags or wrapping the garbage in several thicknesses of newspaper
- placing the garbage outside the home and putting the bags in plastic or metal garbage containers
- wearing disposable gloves if there are open cuts or sores on hands
- holding equipment and linens away from uniform
- not shaking linens which helps prevent the movement of dust.
- cleaning from the cleanest area to the dirtiest (this prevents soiling a clean area)
- cleaning away from the body and uniform (dusting, brushing, or wiping toward oneself transmits microorganisms to the skin, hair, and uniform)
- pouring contaminated liquids directly into sinks or toilets.

- avoid splashing contaminated liquids onto other areas
- not sitting on the client's bed if the client has an infection, to prevent picking up microorganisms and carrying them to the next surface
- wearing disposable gloves during contact with the client's body fluids when giving enemas, cleaning the client's genital area, handling vomitus, and giving mouth care
- wearing a disposable apron when in contact with the client's body fluids

REVIEW QUESTIONS

1. A safe environment is defined as:

2. Two sensory disabilities that effect the elderly client's safety are:
   a.
   b.

3. The five rights for safety in taking medications are:
   a. The right _____
   b. The right _____
   c. The right _____
   d. The right _____
   e. The right _____

4. Who does the Admission Safety Assessment of the client and the home?
   a. physician
   b. risk manager
   c. nurse
   d. HCA

5. Which of the following are common safety hazards?
   a. wet floors
   b. damaged wiring
   c. poisons
   d. cluttered hallways
   e. all of the above

6. Which of the following is NOT an HCA responsibility?
   a. safe storage of medications
   b. administering medications
   c. assisting the client with medications
   d. measuring medications

7. True or False? If more than one person in a household is taking medications, the medications should be placed in separate rooms.
8. True or False? Old medications should not be flushed down the toilet.
9. True or False? The HCA should know his or her limitations in emergency situations.
10. True or False? It is never acceptable to cover the client's face with a damp cloth when escaping a smoke-filled room.
11. True or False? The CDC has developed new universal precautions titled standard precautions.
12. True or False? The HCA can lower the risk of transmission of pathogens by using proper handwashing procedures.
13. Unscramble the following important word from the chapter: fnoniceti _____

CHAPTER 10

Abuse

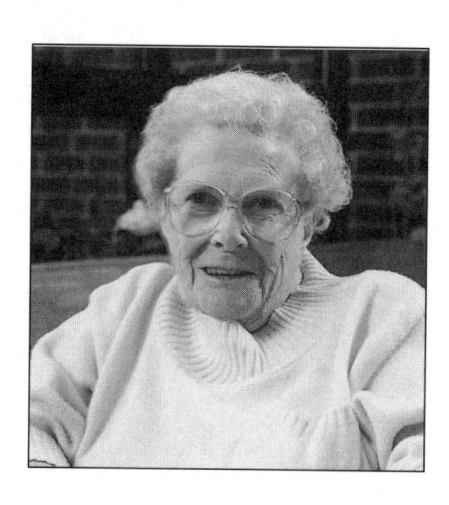

OBJECTIVES

Upon reading this chapter and completing the review questions, the home care aide should be able to:
1. Define the term abuse.
2. Identify six types of abuse and/or neglect.
3. Identify factors contributing to adult abuse.
4. Identify physical indicators of adult abuse, neglect, and exploitation.

KEY TERMS

abuse
exploitation
intervention
self-abuse

INTRODUCTION

Many elderly persons live rich and productive lives with positive relationships with their children and friends. Others are severely disabled, and live in institutions. Twice that number live with, and are dependent on, their children or siblings. Those elderly persons who are dependent are often a physical, financial, and emotional strain on those who care for them. Caring for a dependent older adult in the home can cost up to twenty-five thousand dollars per year. Custodial care is not a Medicare reimbursable service and is rarely covered by other health insurance policies. With these two factors common in our society, the 1990s have seen an increase in the neglect and **abuse** of the elderly population.

Abuse is defined as the nonaccidental infliction of physical pain or injury or any persistent course of conduct intended to produce or result in mental or emotional distress. Severe neglect and severe physical abuse cause great distress and pain and can lead to injury or death. Figure 10–1 shows a client who may have been abused.

Clients not fully able to care for themselves are an easy target for abuse. This abuse can be inflicted by untrained, frustrated, or overburdened family members or by those who deliberately harm others for their own gain. Clients with AD are particularly prone to abuse as their families are under added stress.

SIX TYPES OF ABUSE

HCAs are in a position to notice signs of abuse or neglect. If either is occurring, whatever is seen should be handled confidentially. Any signs or suspicions of abuse should be reported to the supervisor immediately.

There are six types of abuse or neglect:

1. *Passive Neglect*—Harm is not intended but occurs because some type of care is not provided. This is usually the result of a caregiver's inability, laziness, or lack of knowledge.
2. *Psychological Abuse*—Harm is caused to the client's feelings or emotional state by demeaning, frightening, humiliating, intimidating, isolating, or insulting remarks, treating the client as a child, or by using verbal aggression.
3. *Material or Financial Abuse*—Stealing, exploiting, or improperly using the money, property, or other assets of the elderly client.

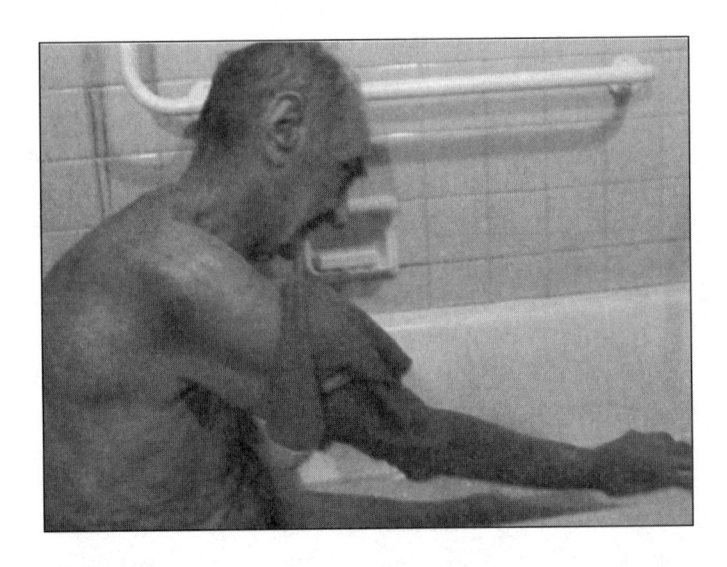

Figure 10–1 The bruise on the client's shoulder is possible evidence of trauma resulting from abuse.

4. *Active Neglect*—The intentional harming of an older person physically or psychologically by withholding needed care. Examples include deliberately leaving a bedridden person alone for lengthy periods or willfully denying the person food, medication, fluids, dentures, or eyeglasses.
5. *Physical Abuse*—The intentional harming of a person physically by means of actions such as slapping, bruising, sexually molesting, cutting, burning, physically restraining, pushing, or shoving.
6. *Self-Abuse* or *Self-Neglect*—Any of the activities mentioned above committed by an older person to himself or herself.

The key for the HCA is to be alert to the physical and mental condition of the client at all times, and to report changes and unusual conditions to the supervisor regularly and promptly.

self-abuse refusing care for oneself

REPORTING ABUSE

The supervisor must be informed of any suspicions the HCA has in order to help identify the proper action to take regarding the reporting of abusive behavior. In order to protect the victim, the situation must be handled carefully; the supervisor and other professionals will become involved if it appears that abuse is taking place.

Helpful Hints: The law states that domestic violence and elderly or child abuse must be reported by healthcare givers. It is punishable by fines and by restraints to work.

The primary reasons for not reporting elder abuse are:
- fear of personal involvement
- lack of evidence that abuse has occurred
- lack of response by authorities
- a generalized belief that reported cases are not satisfactorily handled

There is a responsibility of health care providers to report suspected cases of abuse, neglect, or **exploitation**. Forty-one states have laws that mandate the reporting of elder abuse. The states protect the health care personnel from civil or criminal liability for the content of the report. Each state has its own laws, and penalties are issued in some states for not reporting abuse.

exploitation to use selfishly or unethically

FACTORS CONTRIBUTING TO ELDER ABUSE

The factors contributing to adult abuse include
- retaliation
- ageism and violence as a way of life
- lack of close family ties
- lack of community resources
- lack of financial resources

- mental and emotional disorders
- unemployment
- history of alcohol and/or drug abuse (by the abused and/or the abuser)
- environmental conditions
- resentment of dependency
- increased life expectancy
- other situational stresses

SIGNS OF ELDER ABUSE

The three main indicators of adult abuse are:

1. Personal factors such as ignorance and emotional disturbance.
2. Interpersonal factors such as unresolved conflicts and lack of gratitude.
3. Situational factors such as the dependent person living with his or her children and their families, thereby causing feelings of frustration and stress to the caregiver.

Physical signs of adult (elderly) abuse, neglect, or exploitation include:

- bruises or welts
- fractures
- burns
- lacerations or abrasions
- mental confusion
- poor personal hygiene
- denial of being in pain
- client is bedbound but it is not related to the disease
- weight loss
- dehydration
- old, unexplained scars
- fearfulness and noncommunicative

Some behavioral signs of abuse occur when the client:

- yells obscenities at others
- threatens self-harm or suicide
- refuses medical care
- shows unrealistic fear or hostility (Figure 10–2)
- shows signs of alcohol and/or drug abuse
- experiences denial of the situation

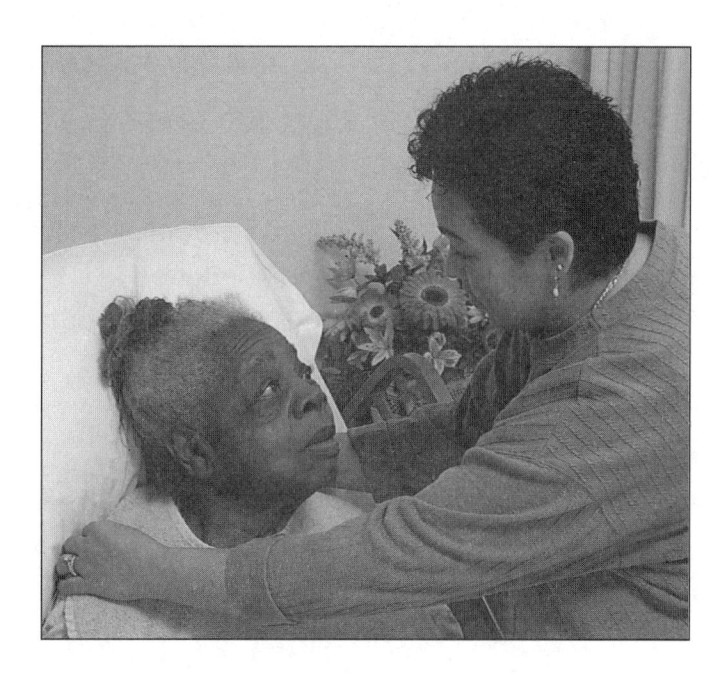

Figure 10–2 A sign of abuse is unexplained fear from the client.

- stops communicating
- is fearful to be alone
- cries excessively
- displays anger at the family
- has a poor self-concept and shows poor self-control
- shows signs of hopelessness

Environmental signs of elder abuse are:

- a dirty house with garbage around
- fleas, mice, and vermin present in the home
- an overcrowded home
- smells of urine or feces
- uncomfortable temperatures
- pets are not well cared for
- empty bottles of liquor or medicine containers lying around the home
- dirty bed sheets that have not been changed
- lack of food in the home
- spoiled food and a dirty refrigerator
- improperly stored food
- lack of special foods for the client's diet
- no available cash
- unusual withdrawals of money from the bank
- complaint of having no money or the family is "stealing money"

Helpful Hints: The client with AD may not be able to verbalize abuse and the HCA should be even more observant for an abusive situation.

SUBSTANCE ABUSE AMONG THE ELDERLY

Substance abuse is a causative factor in elder abuse and alcohol abuse is a major health problem. The third most common mental disorder in elderly men is alcoholism. Some signs the HCA should watch for in clients that may indicate alcoholism are:

- poor personal hygiene
- nutritional problems (weight loss)
- neglect of home
- depression
- suicidal ideas
- repeated falls
- flushed face
- tremors
- extreme fatigue
- incontinence
- withdrawal

HCAs should discuss any suspected substance abuse with the supervisor so that the physician can be notified and orders for **intervention** and referral given. The HCA should look and listen for signs of abuse (see Figure 10–3).

intervention action taken to make a change

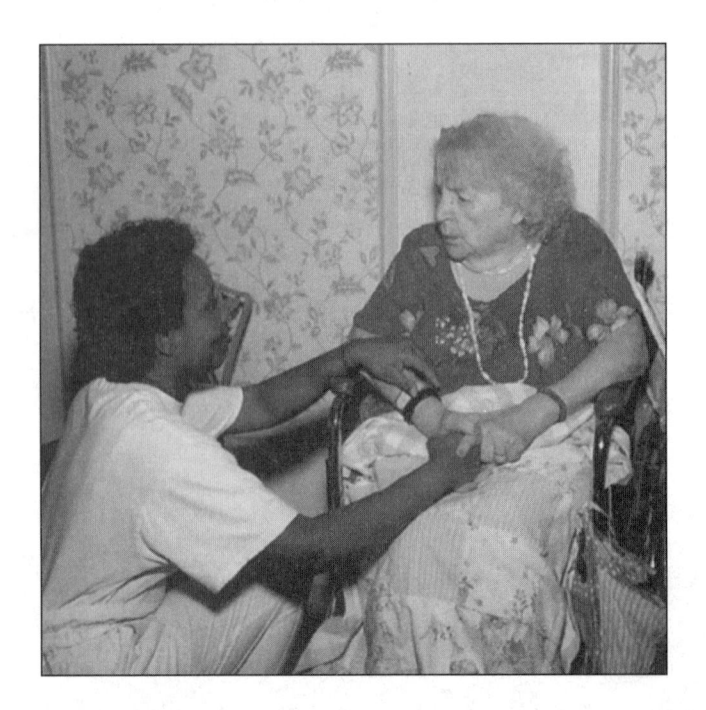

Figure 10–3 HCAs should watch and listen for signs of abuse.

PREVENTION

Some suggestions to give to patients to prevent abuse and maintain independence are:

- keep a network of friends and activities as long as possible
- participate in community activities
- have a "buddy system" with a friend outside of the family and communicate weekly
- make and keep personal care appointments such as with the dentist or a hairdresser
- invite guests to the home frequently
- maintain your own telephone
- be neat and organized
- do not leave valuables around
- do not give up financial control unless absolutely necessary

REVIEW QUESTIONS

State the type of abuse for each of the following situations:

1. A daughter helps her elderly mother by cashing, depositing, and managing all of her income. All purchases and household bills are made for the mother by her daughter using the mother's checkbook. The daughter, unfortunately, paid her own bills from her mother's account. _____

2. A wife cares for her overweight husband at home after a heart attack. A hospital bed was purchased but the wife was never instructed to turn the patient or give him skin care. She and a neighbor discovered, after several weeks, that he had developed three large bedsores. _____

3. A couple cared for the wife's elderly mother in their home. The patient was very confused and constantly caused disruptions, so her bedroom was cleared and she was locked in day and night. The couple insisted they did the best they could. The mother was moved to a nursing home, but the couple refused to pay the bill. _____

4. A daughter, after her divorce, asked her elderly mother to move in with her. The daughter began to date and was away many times during the evening hours. The daughter began to resent the mother's verbal concerns. Excessive name-calling and threats to the mother began. The mother ran away and was returned by the police three days later in a frightened state. _____

5. An alcoholic son lived with his elderly, sick, and obese mother in her home. She was hospitalized for fractures of the hip and jaw and bruises on her face and body. The neighbors complained that the son did not allow his mother to leave the house. She died shortly thereafter. Autopsy reports showed regular beatings had taken place. _____

6. Which of the following are possible signs of abuse in the elderly?
    a. no access to bank account
    b. pressure sores
    c. poor hygiene
    d. fearfulness
    e. all of the above
7. Behavioral signs of elder abuse include:
    a. bruises and welts
    b. crying and depression
    c. fearfulness
    d. burns
8. True or False? HCAs can make a difference in helping the client to maintain his or her independence.
9. True or False? The HCA is required by law to report suspected abuse.
10. True or False? A sign of potential abuse is garbage left around the home and the family pet are not well cared for.
11. Unscramble the following key term from the chapter: rontntivieen _____

CHAPTER 11

Psychosocial Influences

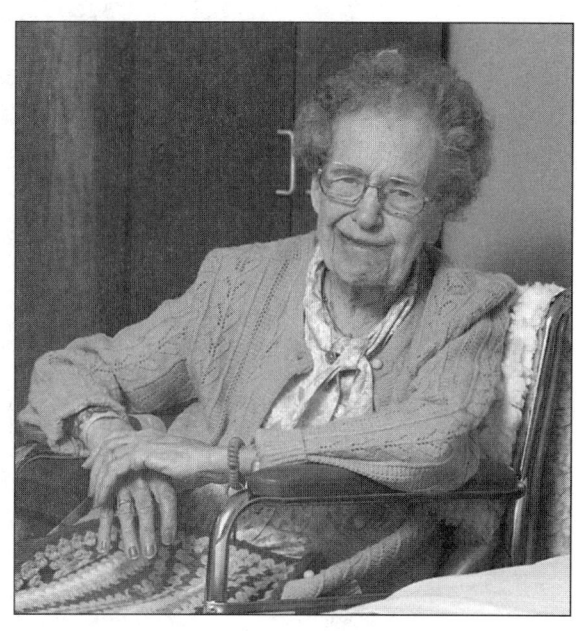

OBJECTIVES

Upon reading this chapter and completing the review questions, the home care aide should be able to:

1. Define psychosocial influences on the client and his or her recovery.
2. Define holistic care of the client with Alzheimer's disease.
3. Understand multicultural differences and human needs.
4. Describe family dynamics and current changes that may effect the client.
5. Be familiar with positive attitudes and HCA codes of behavior.
6. Understand the communication process, especially with the elderly.

KEY TERMS

advocate
confidentiality
culture
disabilities

family dynamics
holistic caring model
impairments
psychosocial

INTRODUCTION

Many of the clients receiving home health care live in a family-structured environment. The psycho (emotional) and social (human interactions) influences on the client affect his or her well-being. The HCA must be aware of these influential factors to better provide the client with a more holistic approach.

THE HOLISTIC MODEL

holistic caring model care based on the belief that humans should be cared for as a "whole" person

The **holistic caring model** considers the whole client including mind, body, spirit, economy, family support, **culture**, and ethics as well as the illness or disease process. and how these factors effect the recovery of the client. Figure 11-1 shows a priest giving the Sacrament of the Sick to a client who is Catholic. The AD client's spiritual side can be easily overlooked and churches and synagogues can be very supportive of families caring for persons with AD.

advocate someone who supports and encourages another person

The HCA serves as a client **advocate** or supporter but there is no way this can occur without understanding the uniqueness and variety of types of clients and families with needs that require special care and concern. Figure 11-2 shows an HCA who is concerned about his client.

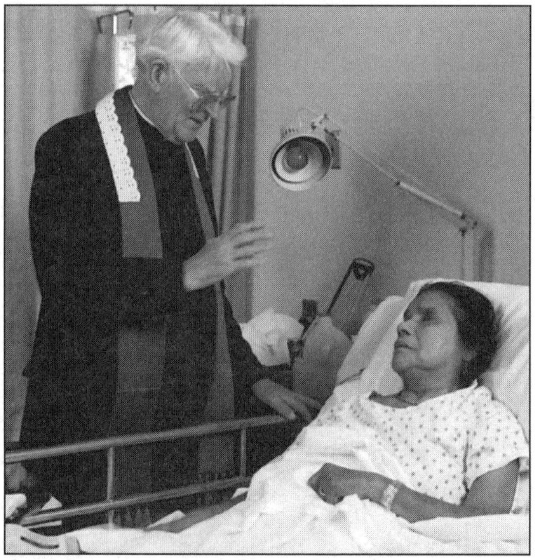

Figure 11-1 The Sacrament of the Sick is administered to a gravely ill Roman Catholic client.

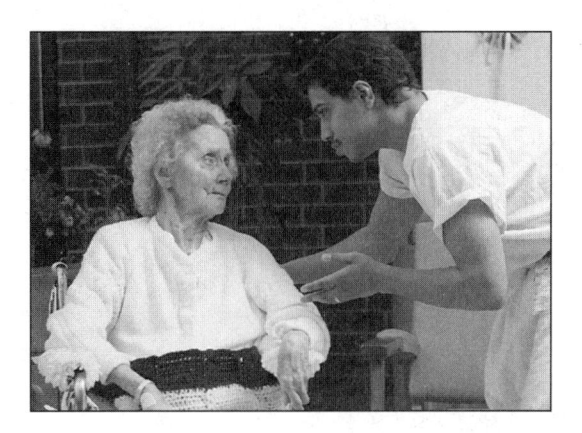

Figure 11-2 The HCA is the client's advocate.

Helpful Hints: If you believe there is a cultural barrier between you and your client or the family, discuss a change of assignment with your supervisor.

The United States has a growing elderly population as well as an increasing multicultural and multiethnic mix. The HCA of the 1990s will be placed in the homes of persons with differences that could effect the level of care or create barriers to HCA/client relationship. Some of the barriers the HCA might see in the home include:

- language differences
- discrimination and distrust
- poverty
- resistance to outside help
- culture bias
- negative attitude toward Western health care
- religious differences
- lack of knowledge of the medical system
- lack of education
- misunderstood family structure

Multicultural differences occur in race, religion, language, dietary habits, gender, age, culture, economic status, and lifestyle. Table 11-1 shows the differences in dietary practices of certain religions.

One area all human beings have in common are their basic needs. A need must be met for a person's well-being. The health caregiver should focus on the client/family's needs first, assess the differences, and merge the two to create a care plan for each individual situation. All human needs are broken down into daily physical needs and daily psychological needs.

Daily physical needs
- food and water
- safety and shelter
- activity and rest
- freedom from pain and discomfort

Table 11–1 Religious dietary practices

Restricted Food	Christian Science	Roman Catholic	Muslim Moslem	Seventh Day Adventist	Some Baptists	Greek Orthodox (on fast days)
Coffee	•			•	•	
Tea	•			•	•	
Alcohol	•		•	•	•	
Pork/pork products			•	•		
Caffeine-containing foods				•		
Diary products						•
All meats		1 hour before communion; Ash Wed., Good Friday		Some groups		•

In addition, the Jewish Orthodox faith:
- forbids the serving of milk and milk products with meat
- forbids cooking of food on the Sabbath
- forbids eating of leavened bread during Passover
- observes specific fast days

Daily psychological needs
- independence and security
- affection and love
- acceptance and social interaction
- trust and dignity
- self-esteem and relationships
- knowledge and achievement

FAMILY DYNAMICS

The family as a unit has changed over the past few decades. The primary family—formerly mother, father and children—is now frequently made up of step-parents, step-children, half-brothers, and half-sisters. The extended family—grandparents, aunts, and uncles—who used to live in the same location, are now scattered over large geographical areas. As travel became easier, families moved to separate parts of the country. Changes seen in the family unit have been the result of many factors such as:

- smaller families
- single-parent families

- divorces and second marriages
- interracial families
- two-career families
- same-sex households
- aging elderly
- baby boomers
- multicultural families
- diversity and blending of ethnic groups

Given all of these factors, the **family dynamics** in the home are also greatly influenced. Other factors contributing to differences in the family that affect the client include:

- increase in medical technology
- growth of new minority groups
- blend of cultures in diet, religion, and customs
- differences in health practices and beliefs
- family structure
- language and communication barriers

Acceptance of these many differences by the health care members is the key to understanding. If, however, the HCA believes the behavior in some way interferes with the client's recovery, it is important to report this suspicion to the supervisor. The stress of having the elderly or a person with AD in the home creates an unusual situation which the HCA should monitor closely.

family dynamics how the family interacts

impairments injury or dysfunction

COMMUNICATION

Of all the factors effecting the relationships and interactions between client/family and the HCA, communication is so important that it requires further discussion. The United States is a melting pot of many cultures with many different languages and various methods of communication. In addition, the client with AD is probably elderly with hearing, speech, and visual **impairments** which can create even more problems in the communication process.

Proper communication is not only what is said but the way in which it is expressed,. It also comprises gestures and facial expressions. A positive and cheerful attitude, which is also professional, promotes a trusting relationship between the HCA and the client.

Some general guidelines to improve communication skills are:

- a calm and supportive attitude
- touch and a caring behavior
- eye contact

- slow and distinct speech with a lowered pitch and tone
- one question asked at a time and plenty of time allowed for a response
- communication that shows respect and dignity to the client
- speaking slowly when conversing with friends and family, each word must be spoken clearly, especially when speaking to someone who is hard of hearing or whose native language is not English
- listening and being patient until the message is completed by the sender, even if that person has a difficult time stating the message; time spent here is time saved later
- not using the words and phrases from different cultures unless the client or family wishes to teach the HCA special words and phrases
- setting up an agreed-upon mode of communication
- reporting and recording of events in simple terms and sentences

Communicating with the elderly is vital to gain information important to the nurse and/or physician. The HCA, however, must remember that the elderly think and speak more slowly than other clients and must not be rushed. Noise and distractions should be kept to a minimum and short, simple words and sentences used. The nurse will determine if the client has impairments such as hearing, visual, or speech problems.

Helpful Hints: The HCA should check the client's care plan for any special considerations in ADLs.

Hearing Impairments

The hearing impaired client presents a special problem for the HCA. The following communication techniques have been broken down into supportive (those that improve the communication process) and nonsupportive (those techniques that make the situation worse) when working with clients who have hearing impairments. Table 11–2 illustrates various hearing impairments and ways the HCA can overcome them.

Table 11–2 Hearing changes and ways to help. (Adapted from Richman & Glantz, 1995)

Hearing Changes	Ways to help
• There is a decline in auditory acuity with age called presbycusis. This age-related hearing loss is usually greater for men than for women. The reason for this decline is not known, but it is suspected that men are exposed to more damaging noise during their lifetimes, possibly resulting from being in the military service or due to the nature of their jobs.	• Any older person may need your help in compensating for hearing loss. While people with visual impairments can compensate by bringing things closer, those with hearing loss cannot similarly compensate. • Speak slowly and clearly, and do not change the topic abruptly. Be sure to face the person at eye level and have light on your face so lipreading is possible. Ask the person what you can do to make hearing easier.

(continues)

Table 11–2 continued

Hearing Changes	Ways to help
• Hearing loss is worse at high frequencies, meaning that some sounds are heard while others are not. Sounds may be distorted, or heard incorrectly, and thus misinterpreted.	• Try to lower your voice rather than allowing your voice to become high or shrill. Women should be especially careful about this. • A sound system used for music, entertainment, or oral presentations should be adjusted so that the bass and lower tones are predominant.
• People with normal hearing have a wide range between the quietest sound they hear to the loudest, which is painful or irritating. For people with hearing loss, this range may be much narrower. Sounds may have to be quite loud to be heard, and sensitivity is increased. If sounds are even a little louder, they may be too loud to be understood or may even be painful.	• Talk to those people with hearing impairments to find out the optimum tone to use. Do not assume that simply making things louder will solve the problem. • Be aware of the fact that noise or music may be irritating and may cause anxiety for persons with hearing loss, even if it has no effect on you. Be especially aware of this situation when you are working with people who are unable to communicate their needs to you. Note signs of anxiety, and try changing noise levels.
• Hearing loss is greater for consonants than for vowels. S, Z, T, F, and G sounds are particularly difficult to discriminate, which causes difficulty in hearing words correctly. Word that are similar can be particularly difficult to discriminate.	• People should be aware of the fact that even if sounds can be heard, they may not always be heard correctly. The suggestions previously mentioned can be followed, in addition, it is helpful to limit the competing stimuli of background noise. Choose a quiet, private place for talking.
• Some hearing deficits can be helped by the use of hearing aids, but these must be worn and adjusted correctly in order to help. They also regularly require new batteries. Some people never learn to use their hearing aids correctly, or they do not get new batteries often enough.	• Older persons can purchase hearing aids from reputable firms and should learn their proper use. Family members or caregivers serving older people also learn how to help adjust or insert the aid or how to change batteries when it is necessary.
• Some hearing deficits cannot be helped by hearing aids, and the person's hearing is so poor that verbal communication is difficult.	• Encourage the use of nonverbal communication such as big smiles, waving, pointing, or demonstrating. Offer opportunities for activity and social interaction that require no spoken communication. For example, cooking and cleaning up can be done in complete silence by two or more people who have good understanding and cooperation. Also, use writing as a form of communication. Those who appear to be very impaired can understand written statements and questions.
• Hearing and following a conversation can take tremendous amounts of effort and energy for someone with hearing loss. Motivation, the context of the environment, and general feelings of well-being and energy can make a difference in the ability to understand verbal communication. Lack of any or all of these may result in apparent "selective hearing."	• We should try to be more tolerant of "selective hearing." This syndrome is often annoying for those who interact with people with hearing loss, but in some cases there may be some legitimate reasons for it to occur. • Provide opportunities for people to participate in activities that are enjoyable but require little conversation—for example, playing cards, doing puzzles, preparing food, and taking walks.
• Depression and paranoid reactions are common among older persons with hearing loss. When they	• Do everything possible to compensate hearing loss and to ensue that people know what is going on and

(continues)

Table 11–2 continued	
Hearing Changes	**Ways to help**
cannot hear what is being said, they may begin to think that people are talking about them and saying negative things. • Hearing is important to more than communication. It is a way of getting signals from the environment, so it also relates to safety.	what is going on and what the conversation is about. If the conversation does not concern them, tell them what the topic is so that they will not feel talked about. • People who work or live with a person with hearing loss should keep this in mind. People ing the community also should realize that when an older person crosses the street, he or she may not hear a car horn.

Supportive Communication Techniques

1. Speak clearly, slowly, in good lighting, and directly facing the hearing impaired client.
2. Get the client's attention before speaking. Do not start to speak abruptly.
3. Lower the pitch of your voice. In addition, tone down telephone bells, doorbells, horns and emergency alarms.
4. Repeat what is said using different words when necessary.
5. Know in which ear the client has better hearing and speak to that side.
6. Recognize that hearing decline is a normal aspect of aging. Convey this understanding through a supportive attitude.
7. Help family members or those who work with older clients become better speakers by pointing out helpful speech habits such as those listed here.

Nonsupportive Communication Techniques

1. Shouting increases nonintelligible sounds and grossly distorts what the client hears.
2. Do not conduct conversations where background noise such as traffic or many persons talking at once interfere with hearing.
3. Do not speak too softly, run words together, or look away from the listener when speaking to a hearing impaired client.
4. Nonsupportive behaviors interfere with lipreading. These include: exaggerated and distorted speech movements by persons trying to help the lipreader, speech that is too rapid, poor lighting on the speaker's face, mustaches that cover the lips, and anything that covers the speaker's mouth such as cigars, pencils, fingers, food, or gum.

Visual Impairments

Working with clients who have visual impairments is another special problem that requires good communication techniques geared for that particular situation. Table 11–3 illustrates visual impairments and ways to overcome them.

Table 11–3 Vision changes and ways to help. (Adapted from Richman & Glantz, 1995)	
Vision Changes	**Ways to help**
• As a person ages, the lens in the eye yellows and thickens. The muscles that control pupil size also weaken. As a result, the older eye requires more light than the younger eye. To see clearly, a 65-year-old eye needs more than twice as much light as a 20-year-old eye.	• Provide adequate lighting. Be aware of poor lighting and that the older person may be unable to see obstacles, read signs, or recognize familiar people when the lighting is poor.
• The lens grows unevenly and becomes striated. The lens tends to refract the light that passes through it, causing glare problems. A small amount of glare that may hardly bother a younger person may cause great difficulties for the older person. Glare also may cause anxiety and inability to concentrate.	• Carefully adjust shades or drapes throughout the day to avoid glare from windows. Avoid shiny surfaces that reflect light. Tabletops, waxed floors, vinyl upholstery, and mirrors may create glare. • Sunglasses, big-brimmed hats, or sunshades may help when clients are outdoors or riding in a car. When clients cannot express themselves, caregivers must watch for signs of anxiety due to glare.
• Changes in the lens make color perception more difficult. Pastel colors (pink, yellow, pale blue) may all look alike. Brown, dark blue, and black may be difficult to identify correctly.	• Do not interpret inability to identify colors as a sign of confusion. • Do not expect older people to use pastels and very dark colors in a color-coding system. Clients should not depend upon color to help them take the correct pill.
• The older eye does not adapt quickly to changes in light levels. Abrupt changes can be hazardous and may cause falls and other accidents.	• Place lights strategically and keep some lights on so that changes in lighting will be more gradual. For example, nightlights in bedrooms will help. • When there is an abrupt change in the light level, an older person should wait until the eyes have adapted before continuing to walk. • Be careful when placing furniture just inside and entryway. An older person who enters a building may bump into things that are just inside the door if his or her eyes have not yet adjusted to the change in lighting.
• Conditions of the eye that cause vision loss are very common among older people. However, most older people are not totally blind and can be taught to use their residual vision. More than half of the severe visual impairments occur in people 65 and over. Legal blindness is most common in this age group. The changes in vision occur slowly, and older people are often unaware of them.	• Older people should have their eyes examined by an ophthalmologist regularly. • Moving closer to things is one of the best ways to see them better. • Extra-large things are easier to see. These include large-print dials, controls, and buttons. • Contrasting colors make things easier to see. For example, doorways can contrast with the wall, wall sides can contrast with the tablecloth, the chair seat can contrast with the floor, and personal items can contrast with a covering on the dresser top. • Avoid clutter. It is difficult to distinguish crowded items. • Do not change the furniture arrangement unless it is necessary; if you do, ensure that older people become familiar with the new layout.

(continues)

Table 11–3 continued

Vision Changes	Ways to help
• Glaucoma is an insidious eye disease that has no noticeable symptoms until irreversible damage is done. It involves a loss of vision due to raised intraocular pressure, which damages the optic nerve. Glaucoma can be controlled and vision loss prevented if it is detected in time.	• There is currently a simple and painless test for glaucoma that older adults should be made aware of. They also should realize the importance of having the test.
• At this time there is no known prevention for cataracts, but they can be successfully treated by the surgical removal of the lens that has become cloudy and opaque. The surgery is usually performed when the vision loss has become severe. The lack of a natural lens in the eye is compensated for by special optical lenses that can be recognized by their thickness and the magnification of the person's eyes behind them.	• If a person has had cataract surgery and wears the special glasses, he or she may still experience some difficulty seeing. The person may need help reading, crossing the street, and doing other things that we assume should be easy. Those wearing the special lenses also may be unsure of themselves and want extra reassurance or assistance. However, people who are very proud may need extra assistance but may refuse to ask for it. Ask people how they might be assisted.
• Cataract glasses make objects seem larger. It is sometimes difficult for an older person to adjust to these distortions. A person wearing cataract glasses also has a blind spot at each side where the glasses cannot provide correction. This situation causes things to appear suddenly—to pop into a person's visual field. There is a new technique of implanting a lens in the eye at the time of surgery that has proven very successful. With implanted lenses, some of the problems of visual field change and size distortions are solved.	• Some people are self-conscious about the fact that the lenses make their eyes appear large and may need reassurance. • To avoid startling someone who wears cataract glasses, approach slowly from the front, rather than the side.
• Macular degeneration is a condition that causes loss of central vision as the macula, the area of the retina responsible for central vision, deteriorates. This condition is neither preventable nor curable. It will not, however, cause total blindness because peripheral vision is not affected. A current method being tested to slow the advance of macular degeneration uses a laser to cauterize the hemorrhaging blood vessels in the retina.	• It may be reassuring to tell the person that he or she will not be totally blind from the disease but will retain peripheral vision. • Low-vision aids such as magnifying glasses can be of some help to those in the less-advanced stages of macular degeneration. • Persons with macular degeneration may seem not to have a severe vision problem. Due to their peripheral vision, they can move around independently without bumping into things and may appear to see quite well. When they talk about their vision problems, other people may not believe them and think they are looking for unnecessary extra help or attention.
• There is some indication that a relationship exists between visual loss and mental function.	• Compensation and correction for vision problems may possibly lead to better mental functioning. It is worth a try.
• Persons who have visual deficits are unable to benefit from the nonverbal feedback important to communication. They cannot see the smiles, frowns, or other facial expressions that are an important part of conversation.	• When conversing with persons who have vision problems, use touch to compensate. For example, holding, squeezing, or patting someone's hand lets the person know where you are and assures the person that you have not walked away.

(continues)

Table 11–3 continued	
Vision Changes	**Ways to help**
• Dining can present special problems for people with visual impairments. These people may have difficulty eating independently or be afraid to dine socially because they might spill or make mistakes. Food that is difficult to see is not appealing.	• For those with low vision, place settings should be uncluttered, colors should contrast, and glare should be limited. A tablecloth or place mat can lessen glare. Someone should name the foods and tell where each is located. Finger foods and snack time should be provided regularly to allow people to feel more comfortable about their ability to eat appropriately.
• Those who have vision problems may be unsure of themselves in social situations and may even be fearful if they are in unfamiliar surroundings and situations.	• Help people with vision problems to look attractive, and reassure them honestly about their appearance. Always explain the layout of a room and describe the people who are present and those who will accompany them to social activities. Do not leave them alone until they have someone they can talk with or until they are touching a table, chair, or wall that will help with their orientation.

The following are some guidelines for such a situation:

1. If the client has glasses, make sure they are clean and that he or she wears them. Also, make sure that glasses are in good repair and fit correctly.
2. Provide adequate lighting at all times. Pools of bright light in darkened areas or variations in light intensity should be avoided.
3. Reduce glare by avoiding shiny surfaces, waxed floors, and exposed light bulbs. Have shades or sheer curtains at windows to reduce glare.
4. Use dishes with brightly colored rims to reduce spills.
5. Use sharply contrasting colors for doors, bedspreads, floors, and walls to help clients find their way and reduce accidents.
6. Provide large print newspapers, magazines, and books.
7. Refer to positions on the face of a clock to help the client locate items on a dinner plate or tray.
8. Ensure that clients with decreased peripheral vision are aware of people or items beside them.
9. Use black telephones with white numerals because they are easier to see.
10. Do not move personal belongings or furniture without the client's knowledge.
11. Use sensory stimulation of sound, touch, and smell consistently.
12. Use large clocks, clocks that chime, and radios to keep the client oriented to time.

13. Obtain talking books and other low-vision AIDS.
14. Ensure that numerals on doors and dials (such as a stove) are large and distinct enough for clients with visual impairments to see or feel.
15. Use magnifying glasses whenever necessary.
16. Give simple instructions and explanations for anything you plan to do such as repositioning the client.
17. Use sunglasses, sunvisors, caps, or hats with brims on rainy days or when there is snow on the ground.
18. Realize elders may have difficulty discerning the difference between greens and blues because of a yellowing of the lenses in the eyes. Assist them to dress appropriately.

Speaking Impairments (Aphasia)

Communicating with clients who have difficulty speaking (aphasia) creates another health care challenge. Clients who have had strokes and are slow to regain their speaking abilities require increased patience on the part of the HCA. There are some important principles to remember in this situation include:

1. When helping a client learning to speak, your rate of speaking should be reduced by prolonging the pauses between words and phrases.
2. The urge to speak louder is great when clients do not seem to understand. Do not yell but speak in your normal voice; emphasize the main ideas and use gestures to help clarify meanings.
3. It is better to ask questions that can be answered with a "yes" or "no" when needing reliable information. If the HCA wants to know what the client had to drink for dinner, it is better to ask "Did you have milk?" instead of "Did you have milk, coffee, or tea?"
4. One of the easiest pitfalls is trying to anticipate the next word the client is going to use and then supply it. Do not supply the word unless the client requests it.
5. Do not talk about a client in his or her presence. It is rude and may also be discouraging to him or her. Aphasic clients, especially, may understand but are unable to express their thoughts and feelings.
6. Be accepting of errors and understand that speech and language will improve given time and proper training.
7. Never speak to adult clients as though they were children. Doing so creates hurt feelings that lead to frustration and depression or feelings of resentment against the speaker. Adult

clients, regardless of their abilities, are not children and do not deserve to be treated as such.

8. Do not attempt to continue tasks that are frustrating to the client for long periods of time. Aphasic clients have a reduced ability to attend to activities for long periods of time and tire quickly. Arrange for short periods of activity and seek improvements in small steps so that some successes are achieved.

9. Discourage clients from staying alone all day. When possible, provide opportunities for interacting with others. This way they will understand that they are accepted and can enjoy life despite their aphasic difficulties.

10. Write down what is to be said if the accuracy of a message is critical or if reinforcement of verbal and nonverbal communication is desired.

11. Give positive reinforcement—both verbal and nonverbal—of the client's progress.

The ultimate goal in communicating with home care clients is to provide the best ongoing care possible. Sometimes this means making changes in care based on the information the HCA sees and hears. The information might simply help provide better care, it could go through the supervisor, or might change the care plan. If the changes are serious enough, the supervisor might speak to the doctor to reevaluate the orders.

STRESSES ON THE ELDERLY CLIENT

The following is a list of factors that can cause stress to the elderly client and may influence his or her recovery. The HCA should be aware of:

- disturbance in sleep patterns
- loss of friends
- loneliness
- fear of illness
- loss of a beloved pet
- decreasing eyesight
- decreasing hearing
- loss of mental abilities
- fear of impending death
- economic losses and concerns
- loss of driver's license
- fear of hospitalization
- illness of a significant other
- feelings of dependency

- wish for more family visits
- less ability to care for oneself
- death of a family member or close friend
- use of assistive devices
- loss of prior social or recreational activities
- regrets
- missing children

CONFIDENTIALITY

confidentiality not taking the client's personal information outside the workplace

Confidentiality means that information about the client and family is personal and should not be repeated to persons outside of the workplace. The HCA must follow the basic guidelines for confidentiality:

- discuss the client's medical and personal facts only with the health care team
- remember that it is the physician's responsibility to give the client medical information.
- do not discuss co-workers or workplace problems with peers or family; go directly to the supervisor.

HCAs should not discuss personal activities in front of the client (see Figure 11–3).

Helpful Hints: Clients in nursing homes or assisted care living facilities (ACLFs) are very curious about other clients and their private lives. Be courteous but firm about not giving personal information about one client to another.

HCA BEHAVIORS AND ATTITUDES

cultures various behavior patterns or life-styles of particular races, nations, or groups of people

HCAs also come from many **cultures** and backgrounds. Each HCA brings his or her ethics and code of behavior to the home which is his or her workplace. These include:

- honesty with peers and clients
- respect of the client's home
- acceptance of differences in families

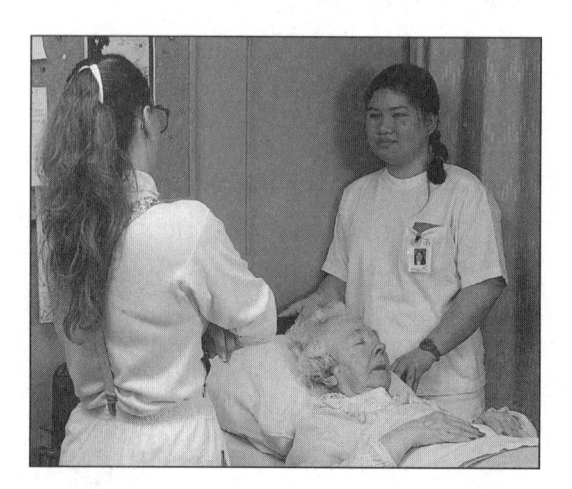

Figure 11–3 HCAs do not discuss personal activities in the presence of the client or family.

- reporting abuse
- caring for yourself and about your appearance
- knowing and respecting the client's rights
- keeping a cheerful and positive attitude
- being dependable and on time
- never leaving the workplace with work unfinished
- not accepting tips or gifts
- knowing the HCA's rights

Positive attitudes that reflect HCAs of the highest level are:

- being cheerful at tasks
- smiling during visits
- happy to do "extras"
- pride in appearance
- following directions well
- empathetic toward the client
- praising even small client participation
- leaving personal problems at home

disabilities permanent conditions that cause physical or mental handicaps or weakness

All persons with **disabilities** should be given the opportunity to live at the highest level of self-care and self-respect and in a safe and healthy environment.

REVIEW QUESTIONS

1. Four barriers to the relationship between the HCA and the client/family are:
   a.
   b.
   c.
   d.
2. Multicultural differences can occur in which areas?
   a. race
   b. religion
   c. language
   d. diet
   e. all of the above
3. Examples of human physical needs are all but which of the following?
   a. food
   b. water
   c. love
   d. rest
4. Which is not a psychological need?

a. safety
b. affection
c. trust
d. dignity

5. Which of the following are examples of factors contributing to differences in families that may affect the client?
   a. language
   b. technology
   c. cultures
   d. baby boomers
6. True or False? The HCA's acceptance of differences is important for the HCA/client relationship.
7. True or False? The HCA may discuss medical information with the family.
8. True or False? Anger is a typical client response to a disability.
9. True or False? Decreasing numbers of friends is a source of stress for the elderly client.
10. True or False? The elderly do not feel stressed or concerned about increasing dependency on others.
11. True or False? Touch can be an effective means of communication.
12. True or False? If the client or family wishes to teach the HCA some cultural phrases, he or she should refuse.
13. Unscramble the following key term from the chapter: mipienmatr _____

Glossary

abuse inflicting physical or mental pain or injury on another person

ADL form a part of the patient's record that documents personal activies of daily living and client behaviors. It is reviewed by regulatory agencies for payment purposes and validates personal care given, along with HCA's home maintenance and nutritional tasks

advocate someone who supports and encourages another person

agitated excitied; to move with an irregular or rapid motion

Alzheimer's disease the main form of senile dementia

Alzheimers's Disease and Related Disorders Association, Inc. founded in 1980 and now has 200 chapters to assist families with understanding of the disease, current research, patient care, and assistance for caregivers

ambulate to walk

appropriate response a response that is suitable for a particular situation

arteriosclerosis a degeneration and hardening of the walls of the arteries, capillaries, or veins due to chronic inflamamation and resulting in fibrous tissue formation

atherosclerosis senile type of arteriosclerosis characterized by degeneration of the walls of arteries

aseptic absence of pathogens

autopsy tissue examination after death

Biofeedback the technique of making unconscious or involuntary bodily processes (such as heartbeat or brain waves) objectively perceptible to the senses (by use of oscilloscopes) in order to manipulate them by concious mental control

blood pressure the pressure of the blood on the walls of the arteries

burnout exhaustion of one's physical or emotional strength

caregiver the person in the home who is responsible for day-to-day client care

cataract a cloudiness of the lens of the eye obstructing vision

catastrophic disasterous

catheter a tube inserted into a bodily passage or cavity usually for injecting or drawing off fluid

central nervous system (CNS) that portion of the nervous system consisting of the brain and spinal cord, including the nerves and organs controlling voluntary actions

cognative relating to, or being conscious of; mental activity such as thinking, remembering, learning, and using language

confidentiality not taking the client's personal information outside the workplace

confused uncertain or unclear mentally

contamination to soil or infect by contact or association

coping skills ability to use learned skills to handle a situation

Creutzfeldt-Jakob disease a rare, transmissible, usually fatal disease, occurring in middle life in which there is a partial degeneration of some body systems accompanied by dementia and wasting of the muscles

culture behavior patterns or life-styles of a particular race, nation or group of people

defecate to discharge feces from the bowels

degenerate deteriorate or ruin permanently

delirium physical condition of short duration with symptoms similar to dementia and/or depression

delusion a false belief despite acceptable facts to the contrary

dementia newer term for group of symptoms referring to a gradual decrease in mental powers and intellectual functions

depression psychiatric disorder of sadness and hopelessness

deteriorte to make or become worse in quality or condition

disability a permanent condition that causes physical or mental handicaps or weakness

disoriented confusion in a sense of identity or location

distraction to cause a person to turn away from a focus or attention

documentation a written account of actions and observations

dysfunctional distrubance or impairment of normal functioning abilities

emaciation extreme thinness

embolus a mass of clotted blood or other formed elements (bubbles of air, calcium fragments, etc.) brought by the blood from a large vessel and forced into a smaller one, thereby obstructing circulation

empathy the experiencing as one's own the feelings of another

exploitation to use selfishly or unethically

family dynamics how the family interacts

fecal impaction a collection of hardened stool in the rectum or sigmoid colon

feces bodily wastes discharged from the intestines

flammable able to catch fire

friction (shearing) tearing of skin from rubbing of other tissue or materials

geriatrics the branch of medicine that treats all problems and conditions pertaining to old age

genetics study of diseases in terms of being inherited or passed from one generation to another

hallucinate an illusion of something that does not exist

HCA care plan a plan developed by the nurse or supervisor as a guide to the care offered, and which contains expected client goals and outcomes

health caregiver the trained health care person caring for the client

High Efficiency Particular Air Mask (HEPA) a special face mask with tiny pores to prevent airborne transmission of disease

holistic caring model care based on the belief that humans should be cared for as a "whole" person

Huntington's disease a disease characterized by chronic progressive chorea and mental deterioriation terminating in dementia

hyperactive excessive or abormally increased activity

hypergylcemia abnormally increased content of glucose in the blood

hypoglycemia abnormally decreased content of glucose in the blood

impairment injury or dysfunction

impulsiveness an arousing of the mind to take unpremediatated action

incontinence lack of control of bladder or bowels

indicators signs that point to specific disorders

infarct an area of coagulation in tissue due to local ischemia (tissue death from lack of oxygen) resulting from obstruction of circulation to the area, most commonly by a thrombus or embolus

infection germs enter the body and cause disease

intervention action taken to make a change

involuntary actions breathing, heart beat and digestion all occur without a person thinking about them

irreversible a condition that cannot be cured

macular degeneration degenerative changes in the macula retinae of the eye, often leaving the person with only peripheral vision

Maslow's hierarchy Based on theory that all humans have basic human needs contained in three levels which must be met: the first level includes food, water, and oxygen; the second level contains safety, protection, structure, and order; the third level comprises psychosocial needs such as sense of accomplishment, self-esteem, and special abilities

meatus an external opening of the uretha on the body surface through which urine is discharged

muteness inability to speak

myelin sheath a fatty, protective, insulating covering of the nerve fibers

nervous system controls all activities of the body and has two parts, the central nervous system and the peripheral nervous system

neurons nerve cells which transmit nerve impulses

orientation to acquaint with an existing situation or environment

pathogen disease-causing microorganisms

paranoia unreal feelings that others are "against" you or will harm you

perineum area between genitals and rectum

peripheral nervous system that portion of the neurons consisting of the nerves and ganglia outside the brain and spinal cord which controls function of smooth muscle tissue, the heart, and the glands

personal protective equipment provides a barrier between the client and the health care worker. When used correctly, PPE provides a barrier that prevents the transfer of pathogens from one person to the other.

pressure sore skin breakdown causing redness to tissue destruction

prevention to slow or stop a potentially hazardous situation

primary caregiver another term for the at-home, everyday caregiver

prognosis probable outcome

psychosocial human interaction

reality here and now—not imagined

respite periods rest from tasks and roles

safe environment an environment in which a person has a very low risk of illness or injury

Schizophrenia a psychotic mental illness that is characterized by a twisted view of the real world by a greatly reduced ability o carry out one's daily tasks and by abnormal ways of thinking, feeling, and behaving

self-abuse refusing care for oneself

self-esteem how a person feels about themselves and their importance and value

senility older term for forgetfulness

spatial pertaining to a space

standard precautions guidelines published by the CDC to prevent the spread of pathogens

stress emotional, physical or mental strain or tension

stress management deliberate attempt to control stress through acceptable techniques of stress reduction

sundowning symptom of AD in which clients tend to wander at dark

support groups persons who have interests or problems in common and offer each other guidance and assistance

syphilis a subacute to chronic infectious disease usually transmitted by sexual contact; progressive and is marked by destructive lesions involving many organs and tissues

technique systematic approach or procedure used to accomplish a task

thrombus a mass of blood el nbements, expecially platelets and fibrin, which causes vascular obstruction at its point of origin

TPR an abbreviation used in medical practice to indicate a person's temperature, pulse rate, and respiratory rate.

transmission-based precautions Centers for Disease Control and Prevention (CDC) recommendations for isolating persons with certain diseases; in addition to standard precautions

validation a communication technique used in moderate to severe Alzheimer's clients to increase his or her self-esteem while affirming feelings such as fear and isolation

visit form a guide for the HCA to document routine and specific duties including treatments, procedueres, and observations (objective, accurate, and legible recording is necessary)

vital signs the pulse rate, respiratory rate, body temperature, and blood presure of a particular client

voice intonation the tone of voice determined by choice of words, calmness or anger

void to empty the bladder; to urinate

voluntary actions muscular actions which are a result of a thinking process

Index

Page numbers followed by *f* or *t* denote figures or tables

A

Abuse, 129–136
   defined, 130
   factors contributing to, 131–132
   prevention, 135
   reporting, 131
   signs of, 132–133
   substance abuse in the elderly, 134
   types of
      active neglect, 131
      material or financial, 130
      passive neglect, 130
      physical, 131
      psychological, 130
      self-abuse/self-neglect, 131
Acetylcholine, 5
Active neglect, 131
Activities, to retain and protect former behaviors, 56–57
ADL sheets, 28, 29*f*
Advocate, 138
Aging, physical and mental signs of normal aging, 8
Agitated, 32
Agitation of the client, appropriate response, 104
AIDS dementia, features and course of, 11*t*
Airborne transmission, 123
Alzheimer's Association, 86
   basic techniques for caring for the client with AD, 100–101
   ways to reduce caregiver stress, 97–98
Alzheimer's disease (AD)
   benign, 16
   caregiving challenges, 21
   degeneration of brain tissue in, 5
   diagnosis of, 5, 16
   disease process, 16
   features and course of, 11*t*
   frequency of, 12
   genetic types, 16
   malignant, 16
   nongenetic types, 16
   problem behaviors/possible solutions, 22*t*
   stage I, 18
   stage II, 18–19
   stage III, 19, 20*f*
   warning signs of, 17
Alzheimer's Disease Related Disorders (ADRD), 16
Aphasia, 148–149
Appropriate responses, 39, 44
Aseptic, 124
Assistive devices, for prevention of skin breakdown, 61, 62*f*, 63
Autopsy, 5

B

Behaviors of the client with AD, 56–57
   problem behaviors and appropriate responses, 101–103*t*, 104–105
   reinforcing positive behavior, 103–104
Benjamin B. Green-Field Library and Resource Center, 88
Bladder training/retraining, 64, 69–75
   areas to focus on, 70–71

assessment sheet, 69–70f
catheter care, 72–75
procedure, 71
Body substance isolation, 123
Bowel training/retraining, 64–68
giving a commercial enema, 64–66
procedure, 68
Brain, 3–5, 3f
BrainLink Materials, 87
Briefs, disposable, 46
Burnout of the caregiver, 99
Burns, first aid for, 117f

C

Calm approach, 100
Caregiver, 89–108
attributes of, 101
basic rules for, 93–94
burnout, 99
care for the caregiver, 96
counseling for the family, 99
defined, 90
health caregiver, 89
impact on the caregiver, 99
levels of basic needs, 107–108
practical suggestions for, 98
primary caregiver, 91
problem behaviors and appropriate responses, 101–103t, 104–105
respite for, 92
role of, 91
stresses on, 92
causes of, 92–93
signs of, 93, 94
stress management techniques, 94–95
ways to reduce, 97–98
techniques for caregiving, 100–101, 105–107
tension relievers, 95
ten ways to help the family, 95–96
the three "Es," 98
tips for, 96–97
Caregiving challenges, 21
Care of the client with AD
activities to retain and preserve former 56–57
communication, 40–44

incontinence, 44–48
nutrition, 53–56
odd and unusual behaviors, 56
personal hygiene, 50–52
sundowning, 48–50
See also Caregiver
Catastrophic reactions of the client
appropriate response to, 105
triggers of, 105
Catheter care
infection, prevention of, 72
procedure, 73–75
Centers for Disease Control (CDC), 122
Cerebellum, 4
Cerebrum, 4
Chemical burns, first aid for, 117f
Children, materials for, about AD, 86–88
Combative client, appropriate response to, 104
"Communicating with the Alzheimer's Client," 82
Communication, 40–44
appropriate responses to problems, 44
assisting the client to communicate, 42
common problems, 40
difficulties, actions/responsibilities of the caregiver, 101t
educating the caregiver, 82–83
facial expressions in, 41
guidelines for, 42
impairments
hearing, 142–144t
supportive techniques, 144
speaking (aphasia), 148–149
visual, 145–147t
guidelines for, 147–148
improving communication skills, 141–142
simple, 100
techniques, 42–43
tips for the caregiver, 41
validation therapy, 78–79
Confidentiality, 150
Confused, 120
Confusion, appropriate response to, 104
Consistency, 100
Constipation, 48
See also Bowel training/retraining
Contact transmission, 123

Coping skills, 86
Creutzfeldt-Jacob, features and course of, 11*t*
Cultures, 150

D

Danger at Rock River: The Neuro Explorers in a Memorable Misadventure, 87
Degenerate, 5
Delirium, 10
Delusions, 43
    actions/responsibilities of the caregiver, 103*t*
    appropriate response to, 104
Depends®, 46
Depression, 9
    appropriate response to, 104
Deteriorate, 26
Diet. *See* Nutrition
Dietary practices, religious, 140*t*
Disabilities, 151
Disease factors, affecting nutrition in the elderly, 53
Diseases requiring transmission-based precautions, 123*f*
Disorientation, appropriate response to, 104
Disoriented, 120
Disposable briefs, 46
Distraction, 43, 100
Documentation
    ADL sheets, 28, 29*f*
    basic rules for, 30–31
    case scenario, 32
    defined, 28
    guidelines for, 28
    HCA care plan, 28, 32, 33*f*, 34
    HCA visit form, 28, 34, 35*f*
    specific to the client with AD, 31
Droplet transmission, 123
Drug resistant, 123
Drugs. *See* Medications

E

Eating factors, affecting nutrition in the elderly, 53
Eating patterns of the client, changes in, actions/responsibilities of the caregiver, 102*t*
Education of client and family, 81–88
    bowel/bladder training, 84
    communication skills, 82–83
    community services and support groups, 86
    coping skills, 86
    diet and nutrition, 83
    follow-up on instructions, 84–85
    handling relationships, 84*f*
    having a caring attitude, 85
    materials for young people, 86–88
    primary goals of, 82
    providing written materials, 82, 83
    safety in the home, 83
    support groups, 84
    visitors, 84–85
Electrical burns, first aid for, 117*f*
Emaciation, 19
Emergency measures in home care, 117–121
    fire safety, 119–121
    first aid for burns, 117*f*
    plans for, 118
    reporting an accident or emergency, 119
    See also Safety
Enemas
    oil-retention, 64
    procedure for giving, 64–66
Exploitation, 131
Eye contact with the client, 100

F

Falls, prevention of, 115, 116*f*
Family counseling, 99
Family dynamics, 140–141
Fecal impaction, 48, 68
Financial abuse, 130
Fire extinguisher, proper use of, 121
Fire safety, 119–121
    elements of combustion, 120*f*
    fire triangle, 120*f*
    using a fire extinguisher, 121
Flammable, 113
Food guide pyramid, 54*f*
Forms. *See* Documentation
Friction (shearing) of the skin, 60

G

Genetics, 16

Geriatrics, 8
Grandpa Doesn't Know It's Me, 86–87

H

Hallucinates, 44
  actions/responsibilities of the caregiver, 103t
  appropriate response to, 104
HCA care plan, 28, 32, 33f, 34
Health caregiver
  defined, 90
  See also Caregiver
Hearing impairments, 142–144t
  supportive techniques, 144
Hiding things, appropriate response to, 104
Higher-efficiency particulate air mask (HEPA), 124
Holistic caring model, 138–140
Home care aide (HCA), roles and functions of
  behaviors and attitudes, 150–151
  documentation
    ADL sheets, 28, 29f
    basic rules for, 30–31
    case scenario, 32
    defined, 28
    guidelines for, 28
    HCA care plan, 28, 32, 33f, 34
    HCA visit form, 28, 34, 35f
    specific to the client with AD, 31
  interaction with health care team, 27f
  observation and reporting
    basic observations, 27–28
    judging the progression of the disease, 26
    safety factors in the home environment, 27
Huntington's, features and course of, 11t

I

ID bracelets, 50
Impairments, 141
Impulsiveness, 26
Incontinence, 19, 44–48
  actions/responsibilities of the caregiver, 102t
  causes of, 45f, 46
  constipation, 48
  defined, 44
  health problems associated with, 46
  skin care guidelines, 46–47
Indicators, 26
Infection
  in clients with catheters, 72
  control
    diseases requiring transmission-based isolation precautions, 124t
    keeping an aseptic environment, 124–126
    medical terms, 123–124
    personal protective equipment (PPE), 122–123
    standard precautions, 122, 123f
    universal precautions, 122
  defined, 122
Intervention, 134
Involuntary actions, 3
Irreversible dementia, 12

J

Just for the Summer, 87

L

Levels of basic needs, 107–108

M

Material abuse, 130
Medications
  abuse of, in the elderly, 134
  five "rights" for safely taking, 117
  safety guidelines for, 116–117
Medulla, 4
Memory disorders
  delirium, 10
  dementia defined, 8
  depression and, 9
  normal aging vs. abnormal aging, 8–9
  senile dementia, 10–12, 11t
    causes of, 11, 12f
    irreversible, 12
    reversible, 11
    symptoms of, 12
  senility, 8
  See also Reality orientation
Multicultural/multiethnic differences, 139,

140*t*
Multi-infarct dementia, features and course of, 11*t*
Muteness, 19
Myelin plaques, 5

N

Needs, levels of basic needs, 107–108
Nervous system
   the brain, 3–5, 3*f*
   central, 4*f*
   defined, 1
   involuntary actions, 3
   neurons, 2, 3*f*
   peripheral, 2*f*
   voluntary actions, 3
Neurofibrillary tangles, 5
Neurons, 2, 3*f*
Nutrition
   client/family education about, 83
   factors affecting, 53
   food guide pyramid, 54*f*
   mealtime, suggestions for, 55–56
   recipes, 54–55
   sample menu, 53–54

P

Pacing, appropriate response to, 104
Paranoia, 19
Parkinson's, features and course of, 11*t*
Passive neglect, 130
Pathogen, 122
Perineum, 71
Peripheral nervous system, 2*f*
Personal hygiene, 50–52
   actions/responsibilities of the caregiver, 103*t*
   guidelines for, 51–52
   preparation for, 51
Personal protective equipment (PPE), 122–123
Physical abuse, 131
Physical needs, 107
Pons, 4
PPE, 122–123
Pressure sores, 60
   See also Skin care
Prevention, 110

Primary caregiver, 91
   See also Caregiver
Problem behaviors/possible solutions, 22*t*
Procedures
   1. skin care and pressure sores, 60–63
   2. giving a commercial enema, 64–66
   3. training and retraining bowels, 68
   4. retraining the bladder, 71
   5. catheter care, 72–75
   6. reality orientation, 76–78
Prognosis, 93
Psychological abuse, 130
Psychological factors, affecting nutrition in the elderly, 53
Psychosocial influences, 138–151
   communication process, 141–149
   daily physical needs, 139
   daily psychological needs, 140
   family dynamics, 140–141
   HCA behaviors and attitudes, 150–151
   the holistic caring model, 138–140
   multicultural/multiethnic differences, 139
   religious dietary practices, 140*t*
   stresses on the elderly, 149–150
Psychosocial needs, 108, 139–140
Punctuality, 101

R

Reality, 76
Reality orientation
   board, 76*f*
   procedure, 77–78
Reassuring gestures, 100
Recipes
   feeling good bars, 54–55
   special high-calorie milk shake, 55
Relationships, learning to handle, 84*f*
Religious dietary practices, 140*t*
Repositioning the client, 63
Reservoir, 123
Respite periods, 92
Restlessness, appropriate response to, 104

S

Safe environment, 110
Safety

in the bathroom, 112, 116f
common hazards in the home, 113, 114f
emergency measures in home care, 117–121
emergency numbers, 111
falls, 115, 116f
general safety measures, 111–112
infection control and, 122–126
in the kitchen, 112–113
maintaining a safe environment, 113
medication guidelines, 116–117
observing for potential risks, 110
reporting an accident or emergency, 119
Safety in the home, 83
Self-abuse, 131
Self-esteem, 97
Self-neglect, 131
Senile dementia, 8
Sexual behavior, improper
actions/responsibilities of the caregiver, 103t
appropriate response to, 104
Shearing (friction) of the skin, 60
Skin care
guidelines, 46–47
procedure, 62–63
repositioning the client, 63
sites of pressure sores, 61
skin breakdown
prevention of, 61, 63
assistive devices for, 61, 62f, 63
stages of, 60
Sleep disturbances, actions/responsibilities of the caregiver, 103t
Social factors, affecting nutrition in the elderly, 53
Someone I Love Has Alzheimer's, 87
Speaking impairments, 148–149
Spinal cord, 4–5
Standard precautions, 122, 123f
Stealing things, appropriate response to, 104
Stresses
on the caregiver
causes of, 92–93
signs of, 93, 94
stress defined, 92
ways to reduce, 97–98
on the elderly, 149–150
Stress management, 94–95
Substance abuse in the elderly, 134

Sundowning, 48–50
actions/responsibilities of the caregiver, 102t
cause of, 49
defined, 18
helpful strategies for, 49–50
ID bracelets, 50
tracer-type beepers, 50
Support groups, 84
Suppositories, 64
Syphilis, features and course of, 11t

T

Talking with Children and Teens About Alzheimer's Disease, 87
Techniques
in communication, 42–43
defined, 40, 100
Toddler toys, uses for, 51
Tracer-type beepers, 50
Transmission-based precautions, 123f

U

Universal precautions, 122

V

Validation therapy, 78–79
Violent actions of the client, appropriate response to, 104–105
Visible, 123
Visit form, 28, 34, 35f
Visitors, information for, 84–85
Visual impairments, 145–147t
guidelines for, 147–148
Voice intonation, 43, 100
Voluntary actions, 3

W

Walking difficulties of the client, actions/responsibilities of the caregiver, 101–102t
Wandering by the client
actions/responsibilities of the caregiver, 102t
appropriate response to, 104

Y

Young adults, materials for, about AD, 86–88